Reflexology
for Children

Kevin and Barbara Kunz

Table of Contents

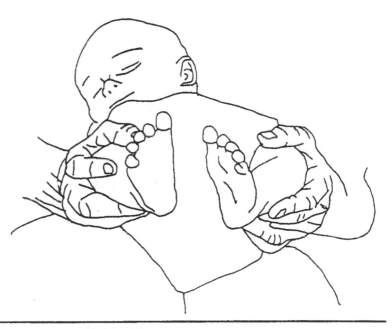

Chapter 1   Reflexology for Children

Some forty years had passed since his mother had worked on his feet when he went to bed every night, but my client had not forgotten. My reflexology work on his feet would put him to sleep in seconds with a smile on his face. He slept so soundly that only his own snoring would interrupt his slumber.

Reflexology serves as a unique tool to maintain or establish a link between adult and child. The stress of growing, the stress of injury, the stress of life — all can be helped by reflexology. Reflexology can be used by parents or a child's significant adults to ease and dissipate the stresses of everyday life in a healthy way.

The use of reflexology's natural touch helps you to build healthy and caring relationships with children. The child gains a sense of worth and well-being knowing that an adult cares and pays attention to his or her needs. As a bonus, the child learns healthful habits to apply throughout life by seeing and doing.

There are many reasons why reflexology benefits children. Throughout this book you will read about stories of success - of adults solving problems with their children using reflexology. Although the problems range from trivial to serious, they serve as examples of significant others applying reflexology technique in a consistent manner to get a result.

Reflexology is the study and practice of applying pressure techniques to pressure sensor reflexes in the feet and hands that influence corresponding parts of the body. The pressure techniques of reflexology relax the pressure sensors, creating relaxation throughout the body.

Millions of people all over the globe have used the techniques of reflexology to make a difference in the health and well-being of another. The popularity of the technique is due to the simple, straightforward method it provides to help others.

The family has played an important role in the development of reflexology. The desire to help family members has launched many people's interest in reflexology and, at times, a career in it. Certainly, the goal of helping a child has provided compelling motivation for parents all over the world to try reflexology.

The goal of this book is to give you the information you need to make an impact on your child's well-being using reflexology's techniques. Whether your goal is to add reflexology to your library of natural health tools, to apply reflexology yourself, or to buy the services of a reflexologist, this book will guide you through your use of reflexology.

Benefits of Reflexology for Children

Parenting children through their injuries, illnesses, chronic conditions, and growing pains provides many challenges. Reflexology works as a tool to address the concerns of every parent in a natural way. Reflexology is a way to show that one cares, to help the child build physical awareness, to provide a nutrient for the body's ongoing development, to create a natural solution to a health problem, to teach self-help to achieve self-reliance, and to use as a special adjunct for special children.

Shows that you care

Touch is a unique form of communication. Studies cite the benefits of hands-on touch to infants, children and even the individual who is applying the program of touch. Use of reflexology technique provides a unique opportunity to get in touch with the significant children in your life.

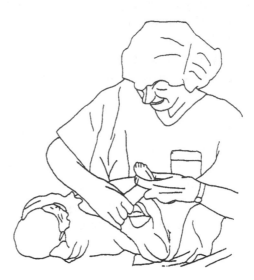

Enduring images of warm, person-to-person experiences emerge from stories about reflexology use with children. One woman is called "Foot" instead of "Aunty" by her two-year-old niece, who remembers and relates to her foot reflexology work. Another woman recounted a childhood memory of foot work to us. Her father would barter with the children on Sunday mornings — if they would work on his feet, he would fix a special breakfast. The fondness with which she told the story spoke volumes. It was a pleasant interlude in the week, creating a closeness between parent and children. A sense of purpose, responsibility, and the family working was reflected in this experience.

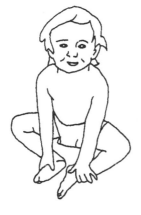

A great-grandmother included a picture of her great-granddaughter with the letter telling us of her reflexology work with the child. She wrote to say that the child was healthy and happy and had not experienced certain hereditary problems. She felt that her reflexology work was the reason. At risk was the child's hearing, and she had a means of addressing her concerns — reflexology's techniques.

One study of reflexology showed that reflexology application provided the family member with an opportunity for interaction with and support of cancer patients. It was the gesture of caring that stood out as a morale booster for both patients and family members. The reflexology techniques established a way for patients to feel the support of loved ones. Also, instead of being unable to show their care and love, reflexology provided a means for family members could demonstrate their feelings.

Helps the child build physical awareness

Adults who seek the services of a reflexologist frequently make comments such as, "My feet hurt"; "I feel that I am under stress all the time"; "I've had a foot injury, operation, and/or foot problem, and I've suddenly become aware of how important my feet are." Actually, many of the body's problems don't happen suddenly. They develop over the years.

The awareness of feet and hands gained as a child experiences reflexology can serve throughout a lifetime. Just as brushing the teeth preserves them, caring for the feet and hands can act as a preventative. The whole body relaxes in response to technique application.

Using reflexology techniques to provide relaxation helps the body break up particular patterns of stress. The stress thus does not accumulate to cause wear and tear on the body. The body becomes aware of any stress before it becomes a problem and makes the needed adjustments. One is provided with a tool to improve quality of life.

The parents of a child awaiting a liver transplant utilized reflexology technique application to help with the complications of the liver disease. For example, the child did not develop the typical yellowed complexion of a liver disease patient. When the reflexologist left town for a vacation, such symptoms started to appear.

Provides nourishment for the body's development

The techniques of reflexology provide a particular nutrient in the body's ongoing development. At each stage of development, messages from sensory organs such as the feet and hands provide important information. This information is vital for the organization of a growing body.

Few go through childhood without bumps and bruises. Pressure to the feet and hands provides key cues in the body's work to heal itself and best adapt to injury and stress. Without an interruption of stress patterns, growth and development can be hampered.

Mothers who have been concerned about their child's growth have utilized reflexology as a tool to maximize the child's full potential. For example, when her daughter's eye was injured in a childhood accident, the mother's concern was that the blinded eye would not track with the other eye. She used the techniques of reflexology to "keep the eye in line."

Georgia Metcalfe, in an article she wrote titled "Treatment at a Touch, How feeling the feet can keep illness at bay," in 1994, recounts one parent's response to concerns about development: " 'Like close to 25 percent of babies in our area, my son Alexander failed to pass his eight-month hearing test.... "Closer examination at an audiology clinic revealed that the eustachian tubes of his middle ear were partially blocked. He is not deaf by any means but his hearing is less than it should be, which could lead to problems in speech development.... " 'Instead of pursuing this course of treatment (traditional medical) I took Alexander to Robert Wynford, a reflexologist who enjoys working with babies although he by no means specialises in them.... " ' Our amateur experiments seem to show that his hearing has improved; for example, he turns around even when we whisper quietly.' "

Creates a natural solution to a health problem

Any child experiences illnesses, injury, or other challenges. The availability of reflexology technique application helps the child cope with life's ups and downs in a better manner.

It has been our experience that reflexology technique application has a natural impact on childhood health concerns. We hear about the concerns from the caring adults: "My child has constant ear infections." "My son is playing football and getting hurt." "My grandson is so overly active that I as his grandmother want to do something." "My daughter has stomach aches all the time."

Some of the concerns take on serious overtones. For example, it is important that newborns defecate within a certain time period. At one hospital, nurses in the nursery call in the "poop" nurse when there is a child with such a problem. She applies reflexology technique to the appropriate area on the infant's feet to cause the child to defecate. Her results were so consistent that when she moved to another ward of the hospital, the nurses would call her to come back to the nursery.

It is not only the illness of a child, however, that tugs at the heartstrings of concerned adults. It is watching a young one go through the experience of illness that prompts many parents to seek to bolster medical care. Reflexology technique application has frequently been utilized in such situations.

For example, ear infection and ear ache are common disorders that take on special concern for parents of toddlers. Infections can create serious permanent hearing and speech problems for young children. Reflexology technique application has given many parents an opportunity to allay anxiety and to seek the best possible outcome for their child.

In several reported instances, concerned parents sought the services of a reflexologist while pursuing standard medical treatment for the child. A British newspaper article states, "Every mother dreads her child going into the hospital. For Kim Badcock the trauma was made even worse because her young son Alistairs' adenoid and ear operations were to be carried out at Christmas.... Alistair came out of the hospital on Christmas Eve, but the next Christmas he would have been back having more grommets put in and would have been having the same operation the following year had Kim, a nurse working in a local GP's surgery, not taken the situation, quite literally, in hand. It was then that she came across an article in the *Daily Mail* on reflexology which said it had been successfully used for the treatment of glue ear.... Although Alistair said his ears felt better after the first session, Kim and David didn't notice any improvement until after his third visit." (Pearson, Deanne, "Reflexology cured my son's glue ear," *Here's Health*, March 1994)

"When Heather Ridenour of Jacksonville was 5, she was plagued by constant ear infections. Her tonsils and adenoids were removed in March, 1981 but the problems persisted. Tubes put into her ears for drainage didn't help and her hearing began to suffer. After three more stays in the hospital and a month of medication, Heather finally got relief:... The cure rested in her feet — through reflexology treatment.... " 'It was unbelievable,' " Mrs. Ridenour said, " 'I would not have believed it had I not been there and seen it. I honestly believe that is what cleared it up.' " (Bunton, Rex, "Reflexology, Practitioners say the foot bone is connected to wellness," Unknown Florida Newspaper, 1982.)

A child can feel isolated and alone when illness strikes, not quite understanding what is going on around him or her. With a touch of reflexology both adult and child are reassured that things are all right, that things will get back to normal, and, most of all, that someone cares.

Provides a lesson in self-reliance

Children's natural curiosity and innate ability to learn create a unique role for reflexology in a child's life. The ability to "play" with one's hands and feet for a benefit does not escape the notice of children.

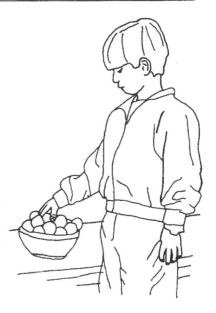

For example, the parents of a five-year-old were driving their son to a birthday party when he insisted they return home. He wanted his golf ball. It wasn't until that moment that the parents realized their son was using a reflexology self-help technique to cope with his migraine headaches. His baby-sitter had placed a bowl of golf balls in the house. She used the golf ball self-help technique to cope with her sinus headaches. He had picked up the golf ball and learned of the technique at her house.

The application of self-help techniques allows the child an opportunity to interact with his or her "owies," as one two-year-old puts it. Some children are too young to convey a message about aches and pains. Few older children are continually in view of a parent or fully report to a parent about every stomach discomfort or fall off a curb. Who better than the child can perceive his or her day-to-day physical ups and downs and address them?

The empowerment of the child to effect his or her body through a tool such as reflexology is beyond measure. How better to engender self-reliance than to give the child a means to communicate with his or her body?

Creates a special adjunct for special children

Reflexology work with special children has evolved. The individual using reflexology to help his or her child has evolved into organizations and schools that utilize reflexology technique application in their programs. One mother of a Downs syndrome child reported to us that reflexology helped with the side effects and problems of the disorder. Several institutions have recently explored the use of reflexology in programs for special children. Several examples exist in the United States, Scotland, China, and India. (See Special Uses for more information.)

An Indian newspaper article cites the use of reflexology at a school for special children. "Mental retardation may not be totally cured, but reflexology is certainly beneficial," asserts Prof. Lissy Jose, (principal of Smithntha Nursery and Technical Training Institute at Inngol in Perumbawoot, India), "It improves their alertness, attention span, and behavioral pattern, apart from improving their general health.... When the mentally retarded are treated using reflexology, their brain improves. Besides the body contact that this brings removes their mental alienation, making them happier. The school utilizes reflexology with its 75 students and as part of the syllabus for special training programs for teachers of the mentally retarded." (Menon, Leslie, *Indian Express*, June 23, 1995, p. 8, "Reflexology - new hope for the mentally retarded," June 23, 1995, p. 8)

Touch as a Nutrient

A mother's touch has a special place in our hearts — and in science as well. Study after study has demonstrated the value of touch. Babies gain weight and sleep better. Touch lowers blood pressure and raises self-esteem. Both physically and psychologically, touch is a nutrient that comforts, reassures, and heals us.

Just as certain vitamins have certain actions on the body, the techniques of reflexology have specific actions on the body. The techniques of reflexology mimic the important function of pressure to the bottoms of the feet. Pressure from the bottoms of the feet helps orient the body. The better one's ability to gather information underfoot, the better one's ability to move through the day.

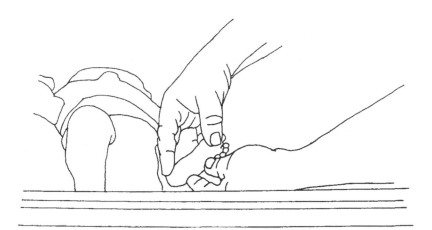

The stimulus of touch evokes specific responses. When the stimulus is pressure and the target is the foot or hand, very specific reflexive actions take place. The unconscious and automatic response of the body links the techniques of reflexology to very specific functions of the body. The application of reflexology's techniques impacts the body's behavior in relationship to homeostasis, the body's natural balancing mechanism. The ability of the child to bounce back from injuries and stress is, thus, enhanced. The role of touch is seen as interacting with the child's development, learning, survival, and stress mechanisms.

Development

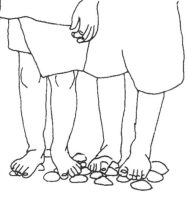

Anyone who has watched an infant grow can appreciate the complexity of learning body positioning, especially in sitting, standing and walking. The waving of hands and feet in the newborn exhibits the beginning of a positioning awareness. The intricacies of sitting up are such that it takes two months for the infant to master it. Standing usually requires six months of experimentation, walking takes nine months, and bowel and bladder control take two years. Even at two years most infants have not perfected all of these tasks. The experimentation with possibilities of positions and movements can be seen throughout childhood. Tricycle and bicycle riding are ventures into balancing. Swinging on playground equipment, jumping rope, and other forms of what is considered "play" are actually an educational process for the body. The awkward teenager is living testimony to the fact that this educational process is at least sixteen to eighteen years in duration.

The nervous system of the body and the muscular system develop as structures able to create function. The football player who hones his or her skills as he or she grows is an example. The feet and hands and their abilities are a part of this process.

Learning by foot and hand

The feet and hands react to shapes. The infant's bottle, the rattle, and toys of all shapes and sizes provide children with the opportunity to learn about their world. So important to development is such activity that it has its own name. Stereognosis literally means the knowledge gained through manipulating objects.

The stimulation received by the hands and feet plays a role in learning the most basic of childhood skills. Picking up a cup or walking up stairs provide practice in shaping the brain and its ability to use objects or move. These are the basic building block skills that enable an adult to write, play the violin or perform any number of activities. Handling shapes builds our consciousness of the world around us and makes us understand that world.

We have all seen the healthy aspects of children at play as they exercise and stimulate their bodies. We have all seen the benefits of sports participation and exercise for children. The benefit is provided by the use of the body for movements and coordination of those movements.

Walking, jumping, running — all call upon the ability of the body to assess the stretch of muscles, the angulation of

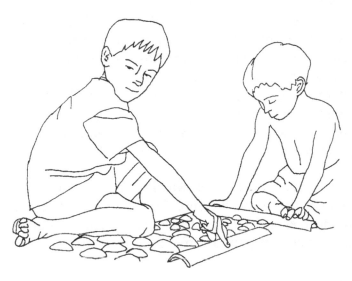

joints, and the pressure to various body parts. The body thus maintains a picture of where it is and what it is doing. Deep pressure to the bottoms of the feet is a specific sensation to which the brain pays particular attention. For example, the absence of pressure to the bottoms of the feet indicates a body position of sitting or lying.

Survival

Anything impinging on the surface of the body needs immediate attention for identification as a possible threat. A pat on the back is different from a poke in the eye, for example. The ability to discriminate the difference between the two is important not only for survival but also the quality of life.

The feet are special sensory receptors keyed to pressure information. Pressure from the bottoms of the feet tells the body that one is standing, that blood sugar is needed in the blood stream, that oxygen is needed for the cells, that certain muscles should be contracted and that others should be relaxed.

15

Such information is crucial to survival. In cases of extreme danger where a reaction of fight or flight is necessary, the feet must stand prepared to participate in either eventuality. This role in survival ties pressure information to the feet and the internal organs. Feet ready to flee need fuel and oxygen from the internal organs to accomplish their purpose. Instant communication is necessary between the feet, the brain, and the rest of the body. Just as one quickly removes a hand from a flame, the body's responses can and do happen instantly.

The everyday activity of walking undergoes the same process within the body. Pressure from the feet helps the body determine fuel and oxygen levels. A demand of running, for example, would require a different level than a slow walking pace.

Stress: The demands of the day

Stress researcher Dr Hans Selye noted the influence of stress to the outside of the body in creating stress on the inside of the body. He observed that burn victims frequently experienced stomach ulcers following their injury. He created a picture of how the body handles stress, including ulcers specifically in response to burns. He found that stress in itself was not a bad thing. It is indeed a part of everyday life. What he did find, however, was that the continuity of stress creates wear and tear within the body.

Russian researchers have found that the continuity of stress can be interrupted. They have created unique methods of using the reflexes to interrupt stress. Researchers have worked with such ideas since the time of Pavlov. The Russians view the reflex as the basic unit of behavior. Within the Russian reflexology model, illness results from improper instructions being sent by the brain to an organ by way of the reflexes. Instead of viewing an illness of the stomach as the result of having a bad stomach, for example, the stomach is viewed as behaving badly because it has been sent the wrong instructions. By interrupting the message in a consistent manner, the organ can learn to behave in a better manner. Better health is the result.

Reflexology as a Special Nutrient

Reflexology includes a basic precept that the application of pressure to the feet creates a specific reaction from the body. Focused pressure application can be used to fashion the response one is seeking. A systematic pattern of applying reflexology's techniques interrupts stress and conditions and teaches the body to behave in a better manner.

The "poop" nurse described earlier actually said to us, "I can make them (the babies) do what I want." As unusual as the statement may seem, this is not too far from the experience of reflexologists. Reflexologists have noticed that their work causes a physical response. The reflexologist-mother who sees that her child is feeling "under the weather," "overly excited," or any number of other states has discovered the same type of response. When traveling by plane, our niece noticed that if she rubbed the ear reflex area on her infant's feet prior to take off or landing, he would not cry or experience the usual pain of such events for infants.

The techniques of reflexology provide a unique nutrient to the body's developmental system. Deep pressure to the foot is a specific form of touch to which the brain pays particular attention. Pressure felt by the feet and hands helps one grow and develop the skills necessary to move about.

As the child grows in stature, he or she organizes internal structures and functions as well. Coordination of the internal organs and the ability to move enables us to perceive and move within our world.

Reflexology technique application provides an exercise of the foot and hand as a part of the body's functions and structures. A mother is, thus, provided with an opportunity to provide a tactile nourishment to her child.

Reflexology technique as a message

What happens when you apply reflexology technique to the foot or hand? Science has not yet formulated a specific answer to the question. It can be said, however that a message is sent. A sensation of pressure is reported to all parts of the body. What happens next is that the message is acted upon. The brain interprets the signal, formulates an appropriate response, and takes an appropriate action.

This activity takes place on a subconscious level, where there are no words to describe what is happening. The importance of such messages has yet to be described by science. A newspaper story gives a clue to the mechanisms at work. Despite the dark curtain of coma, a message got through:

"The sixth-grade graduation ceremony was so important to Esmerelda Pena that she dragged her mother to buy fancy pearl-colored shoes to match a new white dress. Then came the unthinkable.... "Esmerelda was just a few feet from the shoe store when a car driven by a suspected drunk driver fleeing police veered onto the sidewalk and struck her. The precocious 12-year-old suffered a critical brain injury, lapsed into a coma, and appeared to be near death. But her teacher Jose Roberto Vasquez never lost hope. Although the nurses said she could not see or hear him, Vasquez took the bus to the hospital twice a day to hold her hand, massage her feet and whisper news of the upcoming graduation.... Fourteen days later Esmerelda awoke." (Tobar, Hector, "Diploma Honors Girl's Recovery, Teacher's Faith," *Los Angeles Times*, June 25, 1993)

General response

In our experience as practitioners, we have seen examples of both a general response to reflexology technique application and a specific one.

What happens to our bodies when pressure is applied to the soles of the feet was illustrated to us in our work with paralyzed individuals. We saw one body part literally speaking to another. When pressure was applied to the foot, the opposite limb moved. Pressure to a particular part of the foot would cause a specific movement in the other foot or opposite hand. As a session progressed, responses of the internal organs would develop. One client would experience intestinal grumbling; another would experience uncontrollable shivering without the sensation of being cold; two would experience a pattern of sweating. The technique application was, apparently, interacting with the body's nervous system in specific ways. Muscles and internal organs responded to the application of pressure to the feet.

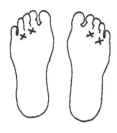

Would you expect to have the same reactions to your work on a child's feet? No, not unless the child had experienced a similar injury. However, the same general things are happening silently with your child when you apply pressure to the feet. Silently, the application of technique is exciting certain organs and inhibiting others. Groups of muscles relax.

The feet and hands provide windows of opportunity to, as it were, reach into the body and communicate with the internal organs and muscular system. The net result of reflexology technique application is a resetting of the body's natural balancing act.

Specific response

Does a reflex area relate to an organ or body part? Does pressure technique applied to the reflex area cause a change in a specific function of the body? The answers to such questions lie in the further research of the work. Any reflexologist, however, would answer yes, quite emphatically, to such questions. Their own experiences have created the core of the belief system.

It is our professional opinion that an explanation for the workings of reflexology exists in the nervous system. We have experienced specific responses by the body as a result of the application of technique to a specific reflex area.

One can imagine the internal messages flying about for our client in the following story. We were paying a visit to a client at home. He met us at the door, said, "I'm so glad you're here," and, literally, pulled us inside. He informed us that he had just eaten a cocktail-sized meatball and that it was lodged in the pyloric valve of his stomach. He was acutely aware of anything having to do with his stomach because he had recently undergone a stomach stapling operation. The operation had reduced the size of his stomach in an effort to limit food intake and, thus, combat morbid obesity. All of us were aware that if a staple broke, he would bleed to death before he could reach the hospital. He led us to his recliner, sat down, and we each began applying reflexology technique to the parts of the feet appropriate to the stomach. Barbara found a soft but distinctive area on the right foot and applied technique for a short amount of time. The client said, "Excuse me," got up, and walked to the bathroom, where he vomited. He came out and proclaimed himself to be just fine.

A distinctive area appeared on the foot in a mirror image location to the pyloric valve in the body. Pressure applied to the foot, in some way, made something happen in another part of the body. The sign of stress in the reflex area was immediately distinctive on the foot. The body's overall response to a stress situation specifically included the foot. (It is particularly intriguing how quickly the body will reflect a response to stress.)

Regulating the internal organs

The answers to questions about how reflexology works have to do with our responses to the world around us. In a situation where fight or flight is necessary, the feet must stand ready to do either.

A dramatic illustration of how the fight or flight response can be triggered from the feet occurred during the course of our practice one day. We were making a house call and Kevin was working on the feet of the husband of the house. Suddenly from the bedroom came the cry, "She's quit breathing." The lady of the house, a seventy-two-year-old invalid who had been diagnosed with multiple strokes and senile dementia, was being cared for by her attendants when she had stopped breathing.

The rescue unit was called. Kevin attempted mouth to mouth resuscitation with no results. He commented, "I don't know CPR (cardio-pulmonary resuscitation). What should I do?" Barbara replied, "Do what you know. Go for the feet." Kevin applied pressure to the adrenal reflex area and the pituitary reflex area. At that point, the woman sat up-right in the wheelchair and began swinging her feet. As Kevin attempted to get the foot pedals out of the way so she would not injure herself, he asked, "Mrs. W., Mrs. W., do you know who I am?" She replied, "Yes, you're a jackass." The others started laughing. They knew she was back; she always talked like that. (Mrs. W. lived another two years.)

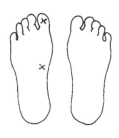

(Note: The pituitary reflex area, the traditional reflexology revival reflex area, is located in the big toe. A primary neuron travels from the big toe to the brain stem, where it synapses for the first time in an area of the brain stem responsible for autonomic control of movement, respiration, and cardiac acceleration.)

A fight or flight response requires the coordination of the feet, hands, and internal organs. For this reason, reflexology technique application provides a means to communicate with the body. While your work may never provide such drama, it will provide you with the opportunity to interact with the body's regulatory system through its tension level.

The foot specializes in sensing the ground underfoot. Pressure to the soles of the feet helps the brain regulate the internal organs. A systematic pattern of applying pressure techniques interrupts stress and conditions and teaches the body to behave in a better manner. Reflexive responses, such as locomotion, alertness, and body awareness can be influenced through reflexology technique application.

Reflexology as a Nutrient for Your Family

The basic tenets of reflexology are simple. In the following chapters of this book, you will learn about them in more detail. While we can describe all sorts of things to you, the particular role you choose for reflexology to play in your child's life is up to you. .

It is perhaps the ultimate use of reflexology to bind the family together. Father Josef Eugster of Taiwan, parish priest and noted reflexologist, reports that he sees mostly family reflexology work practiced in Taiwan rather than professional work. The reflexology work serves to bring the family together.

Use of bodywork techniques by families in the Far East is a tradition that has served another purpose as well. The family utilizes the bodywork technique as a means of maintaining the health of the family unit. In olden days, the purpose was to keep family members working at physical, farm-life tasks. The tradition persists today even with a more urban population.

As you will see in the next chapter, the family that uses reflexology together, stays healthy together.

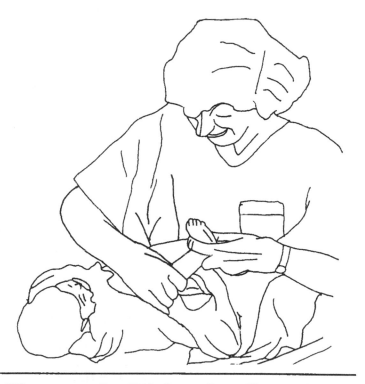

Chapter 2   Using Reflexology

There are many uses for reflexology. For some, reflexology offers the opportunity to spend special time with a child. For others, reflexology provides potential help for a problem. For still others, reflexology offers a full range of such uses.

Jane, for example, was the mother of two teenagers, with health problems herself. She saw professional reflexologists (us), utilized self-help reflexology techniques, and extended her use of reflexology to her daughters. She brought them in occasionally for a reflexology session as a preventive measure. Jane and family graduated as clients and became self-sufficient users of reflexology's ideas. We were happy to educate them to the uses of self-health reflexology and happy to see them launched onto their own lifestyle use. They were happy with a new tool that could be used in a myriad of ways.

Jane's successful use of reflexology for her family paid of in many ways. She improved her own health and that of her daughters. The family's quality of life was enhanced with low-cost, simple reflexology techniques. The family's resources of time, money, and effort were allocated to achieve a sense of well-being and control over their own health.

Whatever your plans for reflexology use, there are a few concepts that will smooth your experience. By considering them, your use of reflexology will be more successful.

Working with Children: Considering the Reflexology Philosophy

It is a basic tenet of reflexology that one's physical being is improvable through a consistently applied program of pressure to the feet and hands. It is a basic premise of reflexology philosophy that one's goal is to help others. Use of reflexology by families has grown into a tradition in countries around the world. This practice has been handed down from generation to generation.

The goals of reflexology dove-tail with the interests of the family. After all, helping a loved one and seeing one's family flourish are great motivations. The ease with which reflexology can be used has made it an ideal tool to achieve an improved quality of life for the entire family.

The basic reflexology approach is simple: Helping others is as easy as working on their feet and hands. Every application of technique has a positive action.

Making it work for you

The successful addition of the reflexology concept to one's family life often follows a general pattern. Jane serves as an example of this pattern. She started small; she kept going; she used the tool of reflexology in a variety of situations; and she chose her moments.

Establish a simple goal

Jane came to see us with a specific goal in mind. Her chronic asthma caused her to awake at three in the morning unable to breathe. She had become desensitized to most medications. A reflexology session would help for a time, but she continued to awake in the middle of the night. We showed her a simple self-help technique which she applied successfully. She reported that she could breathe again within three minutes of technique application. She was pleased to be in control of her body again. Thus fortified by results, Jane focused on her goal and applied pressure technique throughout the day. Soon, she was sleeping through the night.

27

Focused goals lead to improved results. Getting results provides the motivation to apply more technique. This opens the possibility of more results.

Be consistent

More that any other quality, regular technique application leads to successful use of reflexology. In our twenty years of practice, we have noticed that it is those who do self-help regularly or see their reflexologist regularly who enjoy the most benefit. They think in terms of any exercise program and the need to be consistent in any exercise program.

Our thirteen-year-old niece was injured in a riding accident. Her fingers were intertwined with the reins when the horse took off. Three fingers were in danger of paralysis or even amputation. She applied self-help reflexology techniques throughout the day during her convalescence. She credits her reflexology work with regaining the function of her fingers.

Recognize the possibilities

The tool of reflexology is used in a variety of situations. To fit reflexology into your family's lifestyle, consider the possibilities of reflexology use and remember to try it.

Jane's routine use of reflexology for her family gave her a versatile tool to use. For example, she called one day to cancel her daughter's appointment. They were, after all, sitting in a hospital casualty department because her daughter was experiencing extreme abdominal distress. Jane later reported to us that she used reflexology techniques to ease her daughter's pain as they waited. For various medical reasons, no pain-killer was administered during the five-hour wait for the diagnosis and the beginning of an appendix operation. Jane drew on her reflexology experience to calculate where to press her daughter's hand to ease the pain.

Time your efforts

Is your goal to interrupt the stress of the moment, the pain of the moment, or to create a relaxing interlude? Or are you seeking to obtain relief from a problem your child is having or to establish a relationship with a child?

Just as a child's behavior is shaped over time, so too is the behavior of the physical body. The tool of reflexology consists of pressure applied for a particular amount of time. To consider how much time and effort will be needed to achieve a result, consider your goal.

To interrupt the stress of the moment, technique is applied for a brief amount of time. To condition a more long-lasting result, technique is applied over time to targeted reflex areas as well as to the whole foot. To create consistent results, consistently apply technique to the whole foot with regular emphasis on particular areas.

Is your goal to impact a health problem that has existed for some time? Keep in mind that more conditioning by pressure technique application will be required over a longer period of time to change the pattern of stress.

Consider not only the quantity of time spent applying reflexology technique, consider also the timing of the experience. The mother mentioned at the beginning of the book chose a quiet time to apply her work to her son's feet. The timing worked to enhance the effects.

In Summary

Jane's and her family's quality of life was improved because Jane recognized the possibilities of reflexology use. When she realized that she could use the tool of reflexology technique to shape the body's behavior, day-to-day life was improved. In three very different situations — an emergency , her own breathing, her daughter's soccer injury — reflexology provided Jane and her family with a possible solution.

Getting Started

Your overall goal with reflexology is to apply pressure techniques to the feet and hands, making the body aware of its tensions, thus prompting a healthful response.

Working with feet and hands

Allow yourself an opportunity to become familiar with the terrain of the foot. A client once said, "I've never really looked at my foot this long, noticing the shape and the feel." Allow yourself an opportunity to become familiar with applying technique to the feet. The simple techniques shown in Chapter 3 will give you some experience while allowing you to develop your skills. This is a physical activity. Just as one does not learn to play the piano overnight, reflexology skills take some practice.

You may find it easier to begin working with hands. They are a more familiar surface for most. Hands are also more easily accessible as a rule.

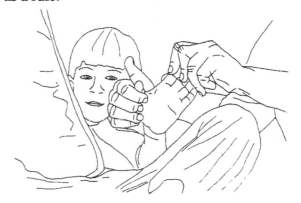

Or you may find it easier to hone your skills by getting familiar with your own hands and feet. Applying self-help techniques develops your technique and assessment skills, as well as giving you the benefit of the work.

Working with children

Applying such theories to your own body is one thing; working with your children is another. Children have minds, feet, and hands of their own. Make it your first goal to get them to accept the touch of hands on feet. Acclimate them to touch so they don't move away, squirm, or find something else to do. You can gradually work on the weak links, working towards a definite goal, maintaining a preventative program — whatever your end goal is. Whatever it is, you are going to have to get them to cooperate.

It is much easier to introduce a young child to reflexology. The younger they are when the acclimation begins, the easier it is to work with them. Birth is best, but before the age of two is very good also. The years from two to five can be a problem because of the squirm factor — a short, short attention span can hamper your efforts to consistently apply reflexology technique. Teenagers trying to establish independence may not want to do what Mom and Dad think is best. This is no reason not to try. Patience can overcome all. There are exceptions to the rule. Children change over the years and even from moment to moment. They may change their minds.

Making it play, not work

Think flexibility and think casual when working with children. While a professional reflexology session with an adult takes place with the adult seated in a recliner, no such formality is needed with children. Casually picking up a child's foot and working with it as he or she sits next to you on the couch makes

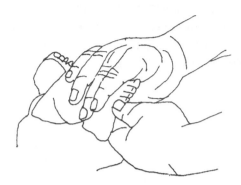

it a part of everyday activity while allowing you to show some attention to the child.

The infant

The feet and hands are natural candidates for playing with any infant. Saying "This little piggy went to market" while pulling or squeezing toes is a staple activity to get an infant's attention. A few presses here and there and some movements and you have a reflexology session that is an extension of a childhood game. Bath time, nap time, while rocking — all present opportunities for your work. A few presses of the foot every day can go a long way.

The toddler

Working with a two-year-old became easy once I discovered the key — turn it into the game the child thinks it is. I adjust my work to the child's speed — I work on the child; she works on me; we both work on the teddy bear.

Allow the young one help in creating the setting. An active two-year-old allowed me to work on her feet for a scant few minutes until she participated in setting the scene. She led me to the refrigerator to get her bottle. She collected her special

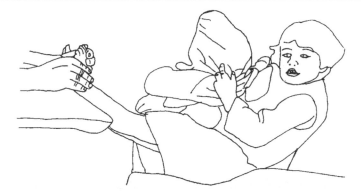

pillow and special blanket, placed them on the floor, and reached her foot up to me in the chair. It worked.

Toddlers will ask questions. Explain your work to them. "You have little owies. We are going to push them out so you have good feelings there instead." The child will thus get involved.

Young children have short attention spans. Until the young child gets acclimated to your work, he or she may cooperate for only a short amount of time only. Stop the session if you need to, but don't be placed in a situation where you are punishing the child during the session. If you need to take further action do so, but don't make it a part of the session. Make it a calming time. If it's not going to work, don't force it.

The older child

Just as there are adults who take an instant liking to work on the feet or hands, there are children who feel the same way. Some children have less affinity towards the activity, but all take notice of what mom and dad do. Children who see parents place a value on reflexology technique application also place a value on it. Also, if the child understands that you are working towards his or her well-being in a specific manner, he or she is more likely to seek out technique application.

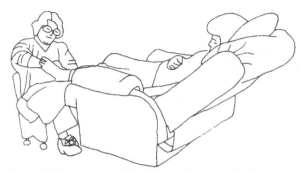

The older child is more likely to sit in a chair opposite an adult to have his or her feet worked. Those under ten have a shorter attention span. Don't expect prolonged sessions. Use dessert techniques as entertainment. (See page 53.) For example, using a dessert to make the foot move very quickly is vastly entertaining to most children (and adults).

The teenager

A teenager who has experienced reflexology from a young age will consider it as a natural part of his or her family life. If you are introducing reflexology work to a teenager, pay attention to what he or she likes — a particular technique, pressure applied to a particular part of the foot, or even achieving a particular goal.

Jane's daughter, for example, injured her ankle playing soccer. She risked missing the last game of her high school career. Reflexology became useful to her when she saw it could be used as a tool for self-help. She applied a self-help technique appropriate for her injured ankle and was able to play in the final game.

Reflexology forms a positive, nonjudgmental form of interaction. It can often grease the wheels of a stressful relationship. You are, after all, both on the same side of the table: their health and well-being is a common goal.

Working with the family group

Consider the competition for your work. I don't compete with a temper tantrum. If one is in progress, my work ceases. I try not to allow competition between family members. It is understood that everybody gets worked on, the same amount of time and we schedule. I don't compete with other activities - video is non-intrusive, jumping up to play with the dog is too much.

Making Reflexology a Part of Family Life

Fitting reflexology into your family's lifestyle may take some thought. Here are some ways that may work.

Monkey see, monkey do

As you can see from the previous stories, children learn reflexology habits from adults. If you do it, they'll do it. Seeing a mother apply self-help techniques, watching mom work on dad, or seeing dad visit a reflexologist — all provide examples of reflexology use for children to observe. The casual addition of reflexology techniques to everyday life makes it more easily accepted into the child's life.

For children who see mom and dad working on each other's feet, it's a question of who wants to be left out? The best way to attract a child to reflexology is to work on a parent. The three-year-old daughter of a client, for example, expects to be treated to a little reflexology before her father. If she has missed her treat, she'll climb into his lap and stick her feet out.

Younger children especially are great mimics. The three-year-old, for example, recreates my reflexology work. She sits

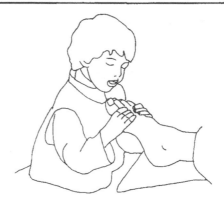

in my lap to work on her father. Sometimes she will push me off the chair so she can sit in it and work on dad's feet. She not only imitates the application of technique, she even studies the foot very seriously.

Setting

Make it a ritual so the child can see a set and setting for reflexology. The above three-year-old has learned that when she sees me at the front door, I am there to work on her father's feet. She helps me move my chair to the den and helps set the chair up. The bedroom was the setting for one mother to work on her son's feet.

Consider the environment you establish for the reflexology work. Anything introduced during your first work (a video playing in the background for example) the child may expect in the future. The association is strong particularly when the reflexology is a pleasing experience. Elements in the surroundings, such as a video, can be a pacifier or a distracting influence. Dogs, doorbells, other children, the telephone, or the television can be distracting to certain reflexology goals. Keep in mind it may be more trouble than it's worth to shut out all distractions.

If your goal is to calm a child or to have a quiet talk with a child, choose a set and setting that provide for quiet time. Many mothers choose to apply reflexology techniques at bedtime because the child is in a calmer state.

Enlisting help

Ideal times may not be always available. Consider enlisting help – mom and dad grandparents, siblings, the nanny, the maid, the baby-sitter – anyone who can apply brief pressure even for a few seconds.

Creating an Enjoyable Experience

Just as you enjoy a relaxing experience, so too do children. Focusing on staying within the child's "comfort zone" with your technique application will create an experience that you and the child will enjoy.

The first rule of creating an enjoyable experience is to be in touch with the child's reaction to your pressure application. Note the effect of your work on the child. **Do not cause pain.** A foot being pulled away from you, tears, or avoidance of reflexology sessions are all potential symptoms of a child's not enjoying the experience.

Your touch and the amount of pressure you use is important. A natural resistance to your technique application will be created if it "hurts bad." Just as Goldilocks was seeking the porridge that was not too hot and not too cold, you will want to find the level of pressure application that is just right for each child. Children have less understanding of "hurt" than adults. Rightly so, their desire is to escape hurt.

Do not fall into the trap of making reflexology work a bone of contention with a child. It is preferable that the child develop a natural affinity for reflexology work. Forcing the child to participate against his or her will is contrary to basic reflexology philosophy. It is the child's body, and it is his or her right to determine what is done or not done to it.

In summary

Whether your use of reflexology is to create a quiet moment, to provide comfort in illness, or to say "I love you," reflexology provides a means of communciation beyond mere words. The use of reflexology creates an opportunity for you to reach out and touch a loved one's life in a positive way. As you will see in the next chapter, learning where and how to apply techniques will focus your efforts.

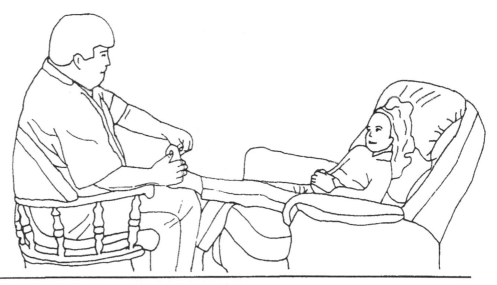

Chapter 3   Foot Reflexology

In this chapter, you will learn how to apply foot reflexology techniques, how to read a foot reflexology chart, and how to assess using foot reflexology.

As described in the previous chapter, Jane knew the tools for the successful use of reflexology. She used pressure to key in on specific areas of the feet and hands. She used her tools in a variety of situations by modifying key elements.

The key elements are

1. How to apply pressure

2. Where to apply pressure

3. When to apply pressure

4. What pattern will best suit your child

The techniques in this chapter are designed to most efficiently and effectively apply pressure techniques to your child's feet. Techniques range from easy to learn / easy to do to more advanced techniques to achieve thorough coverage.

The chart section is designed to help you locate areas of interest on the feet and hands. These areas serve as targets for systematic technique application.

Techniques

To consider the application of pressure techniques to the feet and hands, be your own guinea pig and try it on yourself.

Grip the webbing between the fingers of your left hand between the tips of the thumb and finger of your right hand. Now press this area. What does it feel like? Do you feel tightness? Do you feel tenderness? Do you feel sharpness from your fingernails?

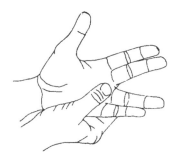

If it feels tight, press it a few times and see if the tightness continues. If it feels tender, press it a few times and see if the sensitivity continues. If you feel your nails, check the angle your nails are contacting the skin. Is it perpendicular and straight in? Try rolling back on your fingertips more towards the flats of the finger.

Your child will be feeling similar things as you apply technique to him or her. In applying techniques, you will want to be sensitive to your child's reaction. Notice your own reaction. When something feels sensitive, you tend to back off and apply less pressure. When you press softly, it feels soft to the touch and relaxing. Your touch as you apply technique is thus an important part of applying pressure. Always remain within your child's comfort zone. (See "Workouts.")

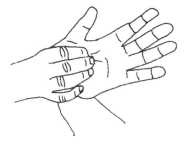

Move your fingers slightly and try applying pressure to another part of the hand. Does it feel differently from the first? Experiment with your hand and see how you feel as you press softly, firmly, deeply, and at a variety of angles.

Experiment on your foot. How does it feel? Compare it to the feeling in your hand. Does your foot feel differently? What adjustments did you have to make in applying technique to the foot versus the hand?

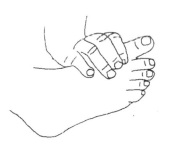

Return to your hands. Apply pressure to one spot as shown. Hold the pressure for fifteen to thirty seconds. Now try holding and applying pressure by squeezing and releasing, squeezing and releasing for fifteen to thirty seconds. Does the area feel differently?

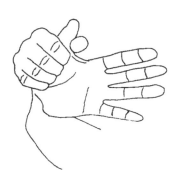

As you can see, pressure is an adjustable part of your reflexology work. The goal is to find the amount of pressure that is right for your child and the situation. To best achieve this goal, communicate with your child regularly, asking how it feels.

Quick and easy techniques

Now that you have tried applying pressure techniques to yourself, try it on someone else. It is a general rule of thumb to begin reflexology lightly. Do not press to your full capacity of strength. Experiment with different strengths of pressure as you explore the techniques.

Single Finger Grip Technique

Seat yourself opposite your volunteer feet so that you are looking at the soles of the feet. Grasp the foot at the base of the toes, as shown on the next page. Now press lightly. Press several times. Increase your pressure. Ask the person how it feels. Get an idea of the person's comfort level. Proceed to a new area and repeat. Work across the foot.

Grasp the side of the foot, as shown. Now press lightly. Press several times. Increase your pressure. Ask the person how it feels. Get an idea of the person's comfort level. Proceed to a new area and repeat. Work across the foot.

Grasp the foot as shown. Feel the fleshy area to the outside of the foot by pressing the finger and thumb together. Proceed to another area and press.

Single Finger Grip Technique

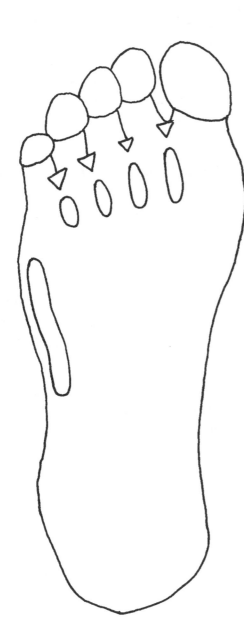

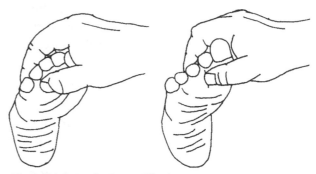

Feel the space between the toes.
Press with the two fingers.

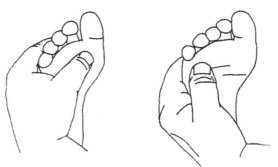

Feel the space between the bones.
Press with the two fingers.

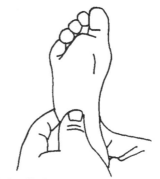

Feel the fleshy area to the outside of the foot.
Press with the two fingers.

Multiple Finger Grip Technique

Seat yourself opposite your volunteer feet so that you are looking at the soles of the feet. Rest your fingertips at the base of the toes. Now, press lightly. Press several times. Be aware of the potential for fingernails to dig into the foot. Roll the finger back so that more of the fingertip makes contact with the foot. Increase your pressure. Ask the person how it feels. Get an idea of the person's comfort level. Proceed to a new area and repeat. Work across the foot.

Position yourself to individual's left hand side. Wrap your hand around the foot as shown. Rest the palm of your right hand on the top of the right foot with the fingers resting on the sole of the foot. Press gently. Then, try pressing a little harder. Ask the person how it feels. Get an idea of the person's comfort level. Proceed to a new area and repeat. Work across the foot.

Position yourself so that you are facing the sole of the foot. Hold the heel of the right foot with your right hand. Rest the fingertips of the left hand at the base of the toes. Now press with your fingertips.

Wrap your hand around the foot, resting your fingers lightly on the top of the foot. Note that your fingertips fit conveniently between the long bones. Now, press lightly. Press several times. Increase your pressure. Ask the person how it feels. Get an idea of the person's comfort level. Proceed to a new area and repeat. Work across the foot.

Multiple Finger Grip Technique

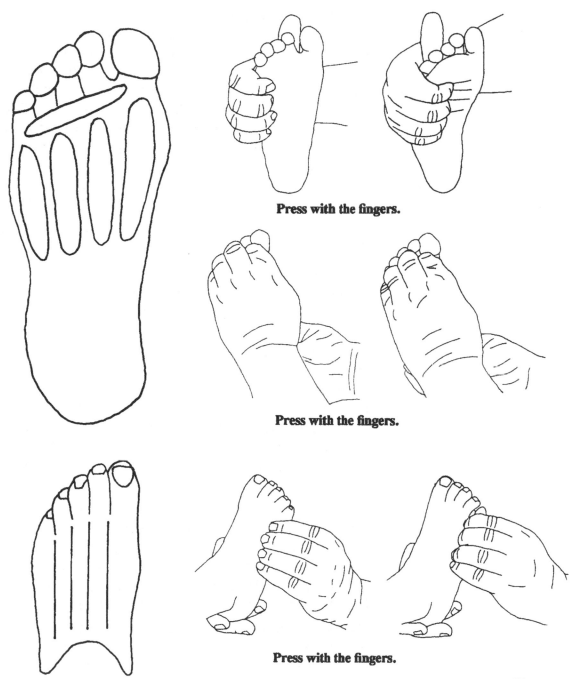

Press with the fingers.

Press with the fingers.

Press with the fingers.

45

Thumb Walking Technique

While the quick and easy techniques serve a particular purpose, a more thorough application of pressure to the foot or hand is achieved with the use of the thumb and finger walking techniques. The techniques described in this chapter are designed to achieve two main goals: efficiency and effectiveness in applying pressure technique to the feet. In reflexology, efficiency is covering a reflex area with the least amount of effort. Effectiveness is hitting the points, being dead on target in every reflex area.

To practice the thumb walking technique, try this exercise:

Step 1: Grasp your thumb at the second joint. Bend and unbend the first joint of your thumb.

Step 2: Rest your hands on your leg. Now bend your thumb at the first joint. Unbend it. Proceed to bend and unbend your thumb, taking small steps forward in direction with each bend-unbend motion.

Step 3: Now rest your fingertips on the surface of the arm. The thumb rests on the underside of the arm. Holding your fingers in place, bend and unbend your thumb on your arm. As you unbend your thumb, take a small step forward. Practice "walking your thumb" in a forward direction. Your fingers stay in place until your hand is stretched uncomfortably. Reposition the fingers and keep them in place as the thumb again "walks" forward.

Step 4: Maintaining the position of your fingers, lower your wrist slightly. Do you notice that your thumb is now exerting more pressure? Now drop your wrist lower. Do you feel even more pressure? The amount of pressure you apply is controlled by lowering or raising the wrist. Leverage is thus created by an interplay of the fingertips, wrist, and thumb tip.

Step 5: As you practice the thumb walking technique on your arm, try to exert a constant, steady pressure. This is most easily achieved by effective use of leverage as described above.

Thumb Walking Technique

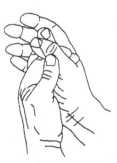

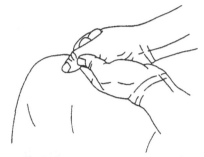

Step 1: Bend and unbend the first joint of the thumb as you hold the second joint.

Step 2: Rest your hands on your leg. Try bending and unbending the thumb. Does it "walk" forward?

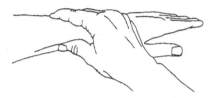

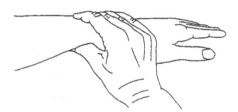

Step 3: Practice thumb walking on your arm. Holding your fingers in place, bend and unbend your thumb on your arm. As you unbend your thumb, move it forward.

Step 4: Practice leverage. Drop your wrist. Do not bend the second joint of your thumb. Do you feel pressure exerted at your thumb tip? Now, try "walking" with your thumb.

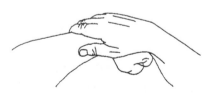

Step 5: Practice applying constant, steady pressure on your arm, hand, or foot to get that feel.

47

Applying thumb walking technique to the feet

Try working with a volunteer pair of feet to become more comfortable with using the thumb walking technique. Give yourself an opportunity to practice. To practice the thumb walking technique on the feet, position yourself facing the sole of the foot.

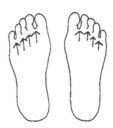

Step 1: Place your hands as shown on the next page. The right hand provides the thumb walking technique and the left hand serves as a holding hand in this example. The left, holding hand steadies the foot and serves to position it to make thumb walking application easier. Here the holding hand pulls the toes back slightly and, thus, positions the foot. A smoother and easier working surface for the thumb results.

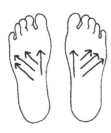

Note that there are troughs between the bones in the ball of the foot. Rest your thumb at the base of a trough. Drop your wrist to create leverage. Now bend and unbend your thumb to move it forward. Think in terms of taking small steps forward and exerting a constant, steady pressure.

Step 2: Follow a straight path, moving the thumb forward, as shown by the arrow. As you finish one path, reposition your thumb, drop your wrist to create pressure, and then move the thumb forward. As you can see from the pattern of arrows, a systematic pattern of thumb walking technique is applied to the feet.

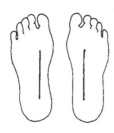

Step 3: Position your hands as shown on the next page. Using the left, holding hand, pull the toes back slightly. Position your thumb on the foot, drop your wrist, and move the thumb forward. As your thumb moves up the foot, note the tendon. Do not apply the full pressure of thumb walking technique to the tendon. Let up slightly with your holding hand so that the foot is not so tightly stretched pulling from the fingertips as pressure is created at the tip of the thumb by raising and lowering the wrist. Change hands. With the right hand holding the toes back, apply the thumb walking technique.

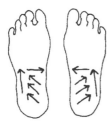

Applying Thumb Walking Technique to the Feet

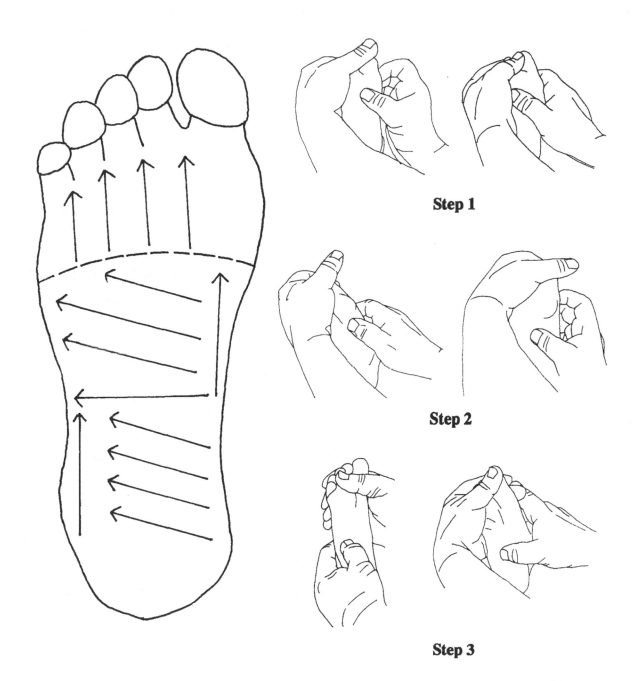

Step 1

Step 2

Step 3

49

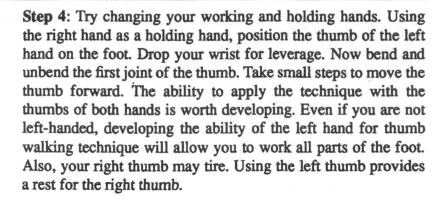

Step 4: Try changing your working and holding hands. Using the right hand as a holding hand, position the thumb of the left hand on the foot. Drop your wrist for leverage. Now bend and unbend the first joint of the thumb. Take small steps to move the thumb forward. The ability to apply the technique with the thumbs of both hands is worth developing. Even if you are not left-handed, developing the ability of the left hand for thumb walking technique will allow you to work all parts of the foot. Also, your right thumb may tire. Using the left thumb provides a rest for the right thumb.

If your thumb becomes tired, you were probably pressing with the thumb rather than using leverage and walking forward with the thumb. Note the illustration on the next page. Only one joint of the thumb moves; the other holds the thumb straight.

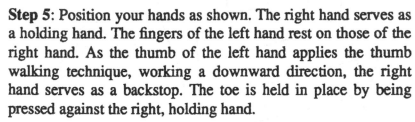

Step 5: Position your hands as shown. The right hand serves as a holding hand. The fingers of the left hand rest on those of the right hand. As the thumb of the left hand applies the thumb walking technique, working a downward direction, the right hand serves as a backstop. The toe is held in place by being pressed against the right, holding hand.

As you move on to walk down the next toe, the holding hand stays in place to serve as a backstop. Try applying the technique to each toe.

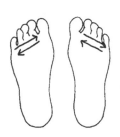

Step 6: Position your hands as shown on the next page. The left hand is the holding hand. It pulls down on the foot to smooth the fleshy base of the toes. The fingers of the right hand rest on top of those of the left hand. With the thumb resting at the base of the toes, move the thumb forward.

Now change hands. The right hand is the holding hand and the left the working hand.

As you move on to walk down the next toe, the holding hand stays in place to serve as a backstop. Try applying the technique to each toe.

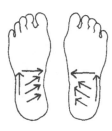
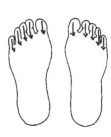

Applying Thumb Walking Technique to the Feet

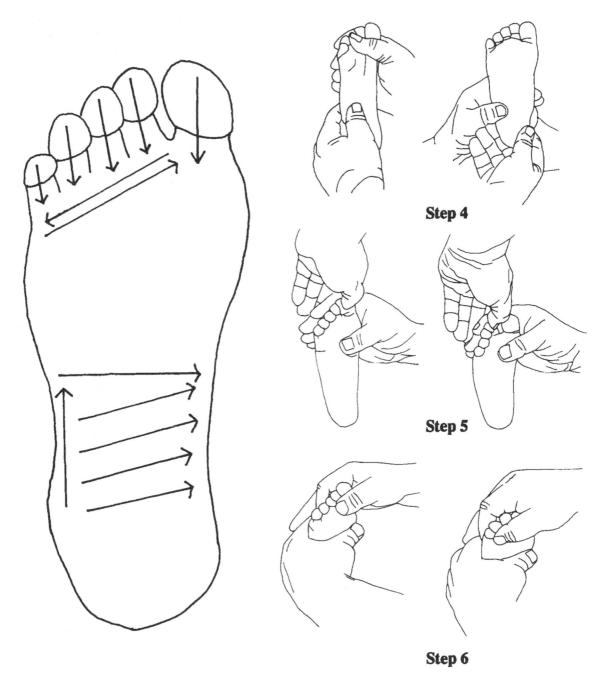

Step 4

Step 5

Step 6

Finger walking technique

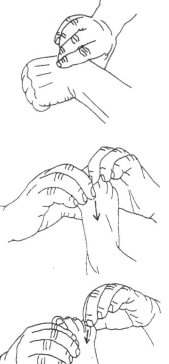

Finger walking is most frequently used on the bony tops and sides of the feet. Either one finger or all fingers work the surface. The basis of the finger walking technique is the bending of the first joint of the finger.

To try this technique, rest your index finger on top of the hand. Now bend and unbend your finger from the first joint. Take small "bites" to create a constant steady pressure.

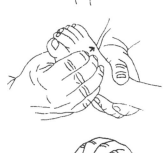

To try the technique on the feet, sit facing the soles of the feet. With the left, holding hand, hold the big toe in place. Rest the thumb of the right, working hand on the ball of the foot. The index finger rests at the base of the big toe. Move the finger forward applying the finger walking technique.

Experiment with finger walking technique on other parts of the foot — down the toes, across the foot, and down the troughs of the foot. In each application, one hand holds the foot to steady it. The thumb of the working hand rests on the sole of the foot.

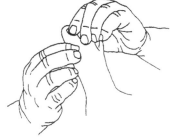

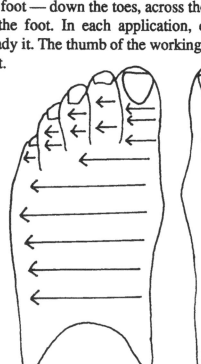

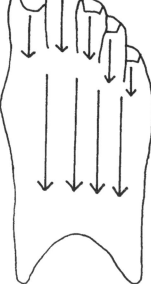

The Desserts

Just as desserts are a favorite part of any child's dinner, the techniques labeled as desserts may become your child's favorites. Application of the techniques is particularly relaxing as the foot is moved in directions new and different to it. As you practice, you will notice that the result of several of the techniques is to move the foot so quickly that it appears to be a blur. Children find it very entertaining to see the foot "disappear" in such a manner.

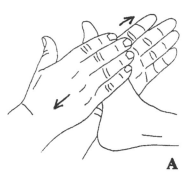

A

The side-to-side technique is a universal favorite. Rest your hands on the sides of the foot as shown. (See A.) Move your right hand and the inside of the foot toward you as your left hand moves the outside of the foot away from you. Now, move your hands rapidly in succession in a piston-like action, one moving forward the other back. The foot is thus moved in a side to side motion.

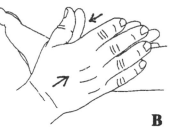

B

The hook-in-the-ankles technique is a variation of the side-to-side technique. The heels of the hands rest where the foot meets the ankle. By moving the hands in a piston-like forward-back motion, the foot is moved rapidly in a side-to-side motion. (See B.)

With the foot-flicking technique, the foot is moved rapidly up and down. Grasp the foot, as shown, with the left, holding hand resting around the ankle. The right, working hand grasps the big toe at its base. The foot is then moved up and down quickly. (See C.)

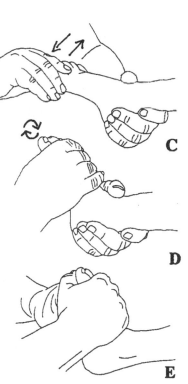

C

D

E

Turning the foot in a circle is a simple yet effective technique. Hold the foot at the ankle with your left hand. Grasp the ball of the foot shown. Now, turn the foot as if you were drawing a circle in the air with the big toe. Do this several times in both a clockwise and a counterclockwise direction. (See D.)

To practice the lung press dessert, grasp the ball of the foot with your right hand as shown. (See E.) Rest the flats of the fingers of your left hand in the ball of the foot. Now press forward with your left hand, then press gently with the right hand. The effect is one of a soft push and squeeze.

Charts and How to Use Them

Consider for a moment touring a new city. Street maps help you to pinpoint your destinations. Charts in reflexology are tour guides to your feet and hands. Charts serve to focus your efforts by helping you to pinpoint locations for technique application.

To best influence specific parts and functions of the body, you will want to target specific parts of the feet and hands with your technique application. Reflexology charts are comprised of (1) a gridlike system of zones, and (2) a mirror image of the body reflected on the feet and hands.

Zones

Zones are utilized in reflexology to link the body and foot. The body is divided into ten zones, one for each toe. To practice this, consider a pain in the body. Note the location of pain "X" in the illustration of the body. Note that "X" lies on the right side of the body. Note that the "X" lies in zone 4 of the body. To find the zone as represented on the foot, consider zone 4 of the right foot.

To influence the body part "X," one applies pressure anywhere along the zone shown as gray. The feet and hands have been found to be particularly effective in providing a location for such influence. The "X" in the body part is thus influenced by applying pressure to the appropriate zone of the foot or hand.

To practice linking the foot to the body, consider sensitivity to the application of pressure to the (1) in the illustration of the foot. Note that the one lies on the left foot in zone 2. Thus, to find the corresponding part of the body, one looks to the left side of the body along zone 2.

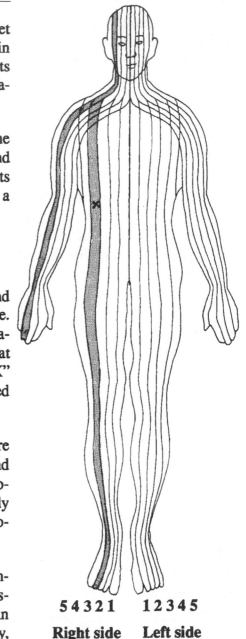

5 4 3 2 1   1 2 3 4 5

Right side   Left side
of body   of body

54

Zones

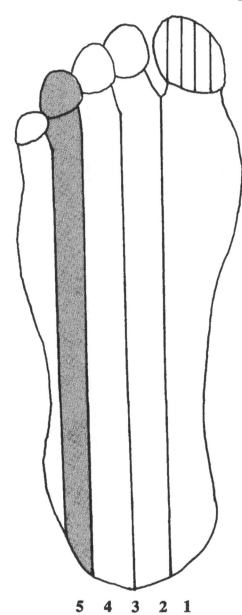
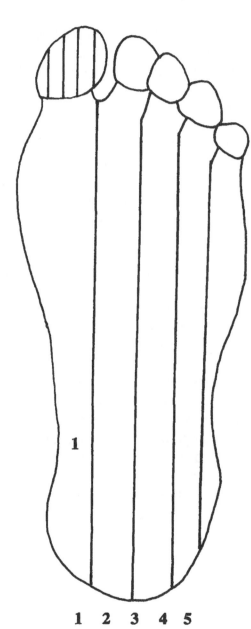

5   4   3   2   1   1   2   3   4   5

Bottom of right foot   **Bottom of left foot**

The mirrored image: lateral zones

To better imagine how the body is reflected on the feet, consider the lateral markers of the body. The lateral markers are (A) the base of the neck, (B) the diaphragm muscle, (C) the waistline, and (D) the base of the pelvis.

These lateral markers are reflected on the feet as well. The lateral markers create lateral zones. Lateral zones serve two functions; one, to further focus efforts to locate a body part on the foot or hand and two, to further efforts to correspond a part of the foot to a part of the body.

To practice linking the body to the foot, consider a pain in the right shoulder. The shoulder lies in the upper portion of the body and to the outside. To find a corresponding part of the foot, look at the upper portion to the outside of the right foot.

This system also is applied to influence a function of the body. For example, a client was experiencing extreme gastric distress and was being driven to the casualty department. It was a sixty-mile drive so she decided to apply reflexology technique to her hand. She was aware of the location for the reflex areas on her hand for the digestive system. She probed until she found the sore spot and then applied pressure.

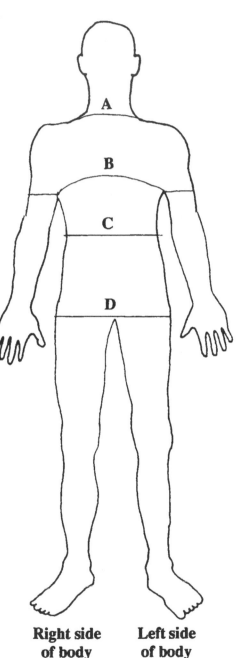

Right side of body   **Left side of body**

The Mirrored Image: Lateral Zones

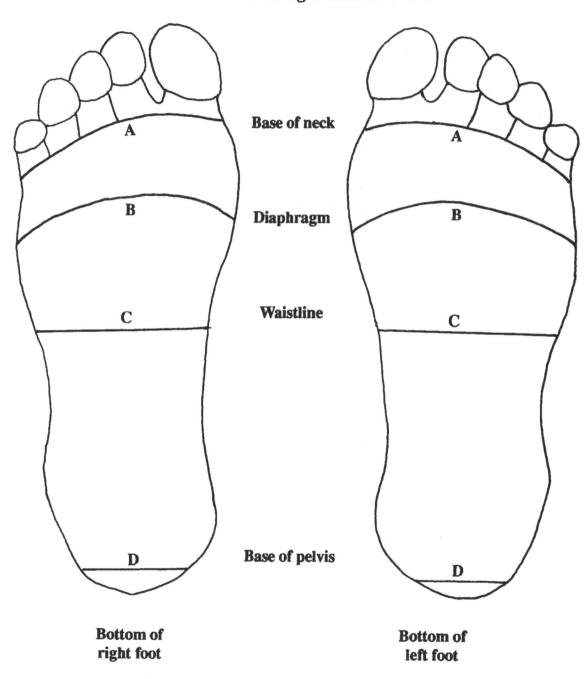

Base of neck

Diaphragm

Waistline

Base of pelvis

Bottom of
right foot

Bottom of
left foot

The mirrored image: longitudinal and lateral zones

The mirrored image of the body on the foot becomes more specific when both longitudinal zones and lateral zones are considered. Just as a map of a city forms a grid, the relationship charts between body and foot form a grid-like pattern. A tool is thus created to correspond a part of the body to the foot and hand and vice versa.

As a practice exercise, look at the illustration. Notice the spot marked "X" where, let's say, there is some pain or injury. By tracing along the appropriate zone into the foot, you can find sensitivity there too.

As a further exercise, visualize the back view of the trunk of the body projected onto the feet. The spine runs down the inside of each foot. The shoulder joint lies to the outside of the foot. The arm extends along the outside of the foot with the elbow falling at the waistline marker. The hips are located in the heel of the foot.

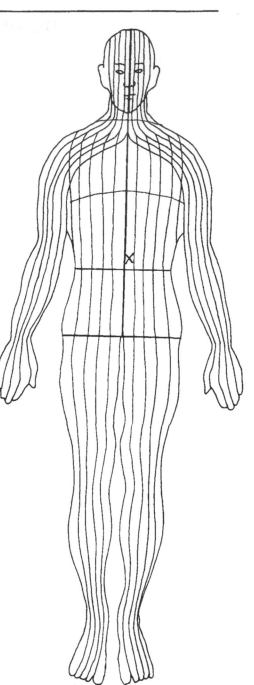

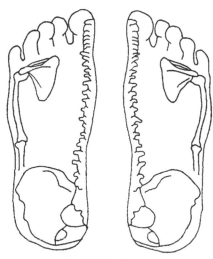

Skeletal system mirrored on the feet

Right side of body   **Left side of body**

The Mirrored Image: Longitudinal and Lateral Zones

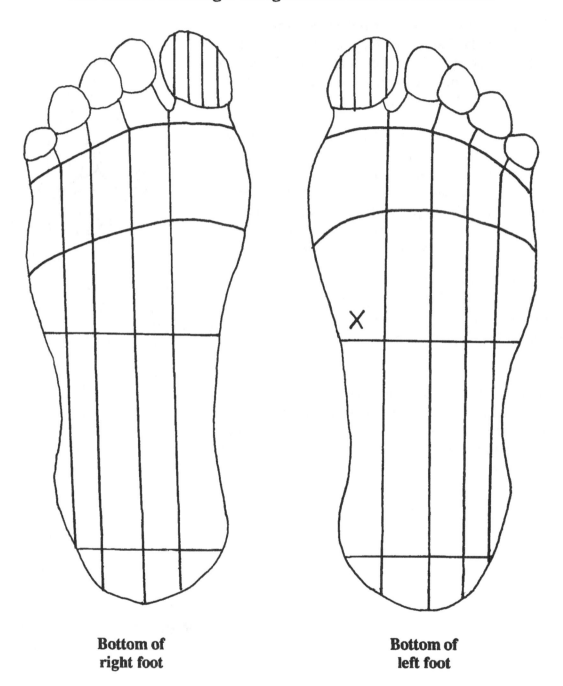

**Bottom of
right foot**

**Bottom of
left foot**

The mirrored image: foot reflex areas

The foot reflexology chart reflects a mirror image of the body on the foot. It is a map of the organs within the gridlike zone system. It is used as a specific tool to focus on specific organs, systems, or functions of the body that may be under stress.

The ability to target one's concern in such a manner has very practical applications; for example, the gentleman in Chapter 1 who met us at the door reporting distress of the pyloric valve of his stomach. Our response to his request for reflexology work was to apply pressure technique to the stomach reflex area. An area of hardness was felt in the stomach reflex area. (See X.)

"Where do we work for cardiac problems?" was the question from a group of nurses from a cardiac care unit of a hospital. We drew their attention to the heart reflex area which lies on the ball of the foot under the big toe of both feet.

As you can see, use of the reflexology chart in this manner is a fast and simple way to locate and work with areas of concern. The simple formula of "finding a sore spot and rubbing it out" has been successful for a myriad of individuals.

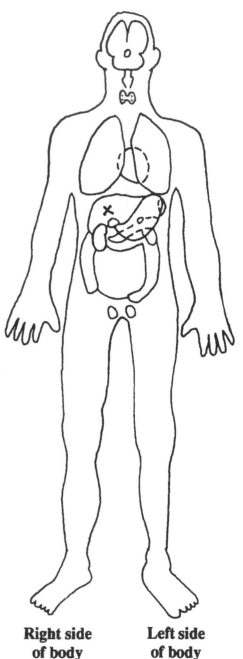

**Right side
of body**   **Left side
of body**

Foot Reflexology Chart

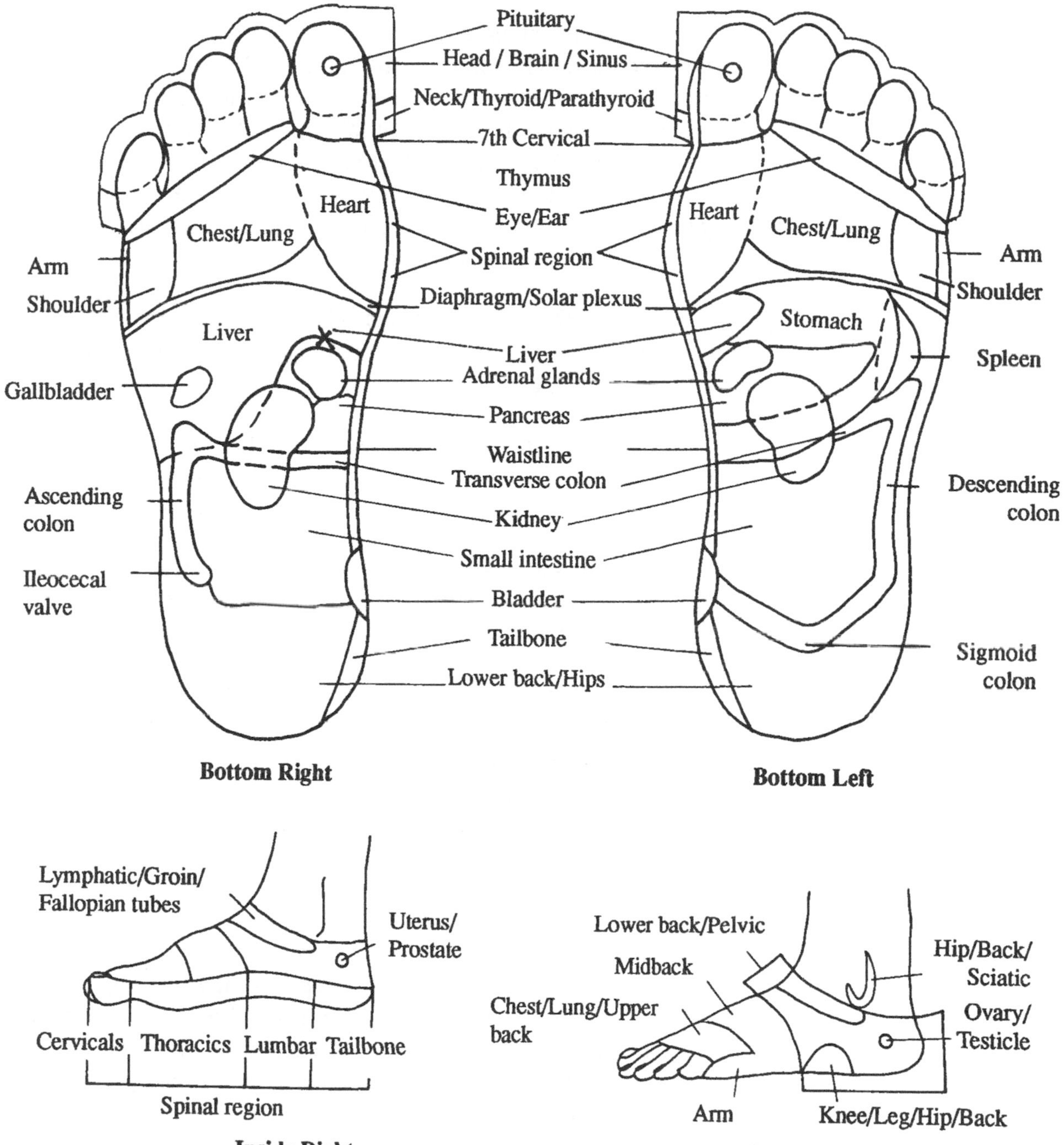

Pituitary

Head / Brain / Sinus

Neck/Thyroid/Parathyroid

7th Cervical

Thymus

Heart — Eye/Ear — Heart

Chest/Lung — Spinal region — Chest/Lung

Arm — Diaphragm/Solar plexus — Arm

Shoulder — Shoulder

Liver — Stomach

Gallbladder — Liver — Spleen

Adrenal glands

Pancreas

Waistline

Ascending colon — Transverse colon — Descending colon

Kidney

Small intestine

Ileocecal valve — Bladder

Tailbone — Sigmoid colon

Lower back/Hips

Bottom Right   **Bottom Left**

Lymphatic/Groin/
Fallopian tubes

Uterus/
Prostate

Lower back/Pelvic

Midback

Hip/Back/
Sciatic

Chest/Lung/Upper
back

Ovary/
Testicle

Cervicals Thoracics Lumbar Tailbone

Spinal region

Arm

Knee/Leg/Hip/Back

Inside Right   **Outside Left**

61

The Whole Foot Workout

Technique applied to the whole foot provides several benefits. The thorough workout can give you a broader frame of reference for your reflexology work. You will be familiar with the feel of the child's foot and can tell that a change in stress level has occurred. You will be develop the ability to feel that change has occurred in response to your work. The whole foot workout gives you an opportunity to compare and contrast the "feel" of one part of the foot to another.

Finally, the whole foot is provided with exercise and relaxation. Working with the entire foot thus provides a more holistic approach in general.

Work on the right foot is illustrated. A full workout includes work on both feet. Illustrations are given of the reflex areas of the left foot which are not common to both feet.

1 Begin your workout by checking to see if there are any areas to be aware of such as, cuts or bruises. Avoid work on these areas. Cover cuts with a bandage to avoid touching them.

2–5 Begin your work with a series of dessert / relaxation techniques. These techniques can be used throughout the session as you wish. Desserts are applied between work on parts of the foot, such as the toes and the ball of the foot. Also, if an area has been sensitive to work, a dessert will help soothe things.

6–9 When working with the toes, the holding hand is important in keeping the toes in an upright position. (6) Note that the big toe is simply held. (7–9) Note that the holding hand serves as a backstop. As pressure is applied, the working thumb presses the toe against the backstop hand. Pressure applied to the toes may create a response of sensitivity from the child. Apply some desserts to soothe the response. Adjust your pressure to match the child's sensitivity.

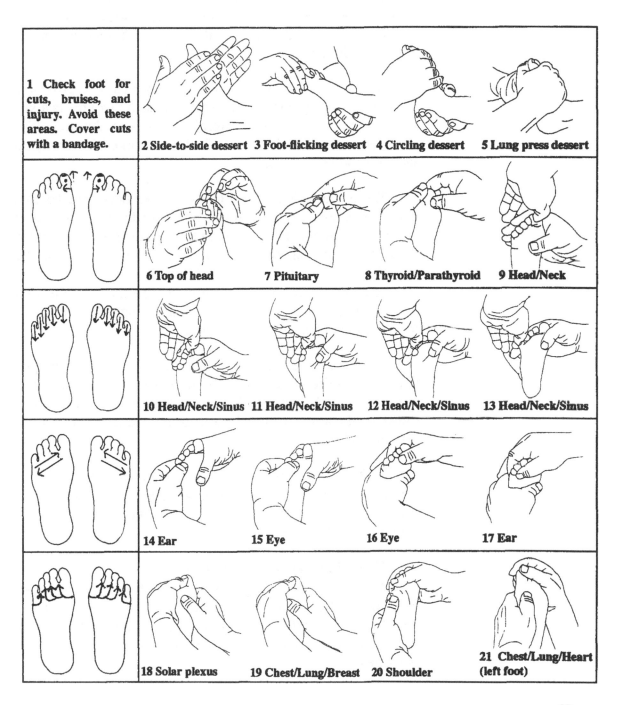

1 Check foot for cuts, bruises, and injury. Avoid these areas. Cover cuts with a bandage.

2 Side-to-side dessert 3 Foot-flicking dessert 4 Circling dessert 5 Lung press dessert

6 Top of head 7 Pituitary 8 Thyroid/Parathyroid 9 Head/Neck

10 Head/Neck/Sinus 11 Head/Neck/Sinus 12 Head/Neck/Sinus 13 Head/Neck/Sinus

14 Ear 15 Eye 16 Eye 17 Ear

18 Solar plexus 19 Chest/Lung/Breast 20 Shoulder 21 Chest/Lung/Heart (left foot)

14–17 The holding hand pulls down on the fleshy ball of the foot. The working thumb is thus provided with a more easily worked surface at the base of the toes. Technique is applied from both directions.

18–21 The holding hand holds the toes back to provide a smoother working surface. The solar plexus reflex area is a key area for relaxation. Make several passes over the area. The shoulder reflex area is most effectively worked by changing working and holding hands.

22–25 The holding hand holds the toes back. The adrenal gland reflex area lies to the inside of the tendon you can feel. It is approximately halfway between the waistline marker and the solar plexus marker. As the working thumb progresses up the foot, follow along the inside of the tendon to best target the adrenal gland reflex area. (Do not work directly on the tendon itself when the foot is pulled taut.) Try applying the technique in the direction indicated by the arrows.

26–29 To more easily apply the thumb walking technique, remember to drop your wrist and establish leverage and then move the thumb forward. Move the thumb in the directions shown by the arrow. Cover the area below the waistline marker systematically.

30–33 Change hands and walk from the other direction. As you work through the foot, note what you feel under your thumb. Does working from one direction feel differently than working from the other?

38–41 Hold the foot steady so that the inside edge is accessible to your working thumb. Cup the heel in your working hand. Begin the technique application toward the back of the heel. Move the working thumb in a forward direction. As you work, reposition your working hand so that the thumb is not over-stretched.

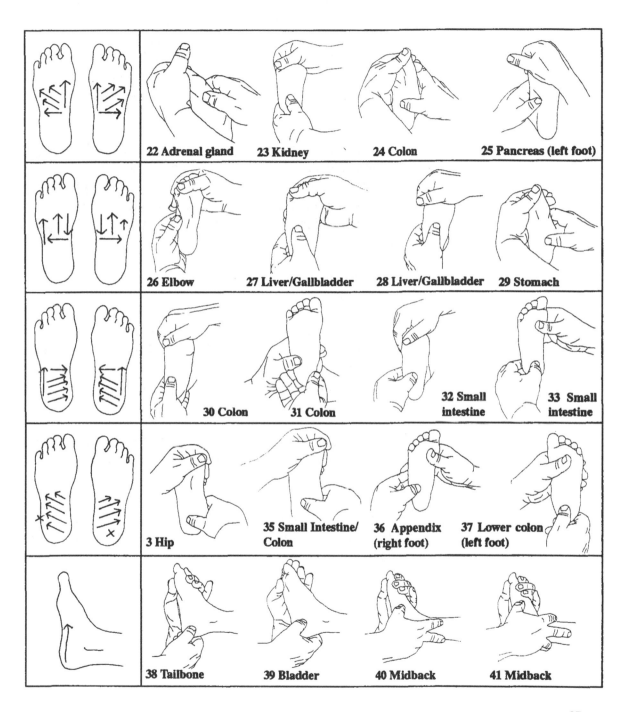

22 Adrenal gland 23 Kidney 24 Colon 25 Pancreas (left foot)

26 Elbow 27 Liver/Gallbladder 28 Liver/Gallbladder 29 Stomach

30 Colon 31 Colon 32 Small intestine 33 Small intestine

3 Hip 35 Small Intestine/Colon 36 Appendix (right foot) 37 Lower colon (left foot)

38 Tailbone 39 Bladder 40 Midback 41 Midback

65

42–44 The holding hand holds the big toe in position for the working thumb. **(45)** Cup the heel, curling the third finger in such a way as to place its tip on the point to be worked. The thumb wraps around the ankle. Now rotate the foot in a counter-clockwise direction several times, drawing circles in the air with the big toe. Next rotate the foot in a clockwise direction several times.

46 Hold the foot in a steady position. The working finger moves across the big toe. **(47)** The big toe is held in place as the finger moves across the base of the toe. **(48)** Multiple fingers move with a finger walking technique across the top of the foot. **(49)** Thumb walking technique is applied where the foot joins the ankle.

50–53 Hold the foot steady and apply finger walking technique to the tops of the toes.

54–57 The holding hand holds the toes apart. The thumb of the working hand is placed on the bottom of the foot. The working finger moves down the trough formed by two of the long bones. Move on to the next trough. Separate the toes with the holding hand.

58 The holding hand cups the heel. The working finger moves around the ankle bone. **(59)** Hold the foot steady and use the thumb walking technique to make several passes through the heel area. **(60)** Note the semi-circular area above the heel. Apply the thumb walking technique in the direction of the arrows. **(61)** Proceed with the thumb walking technique up the outside of the foot.

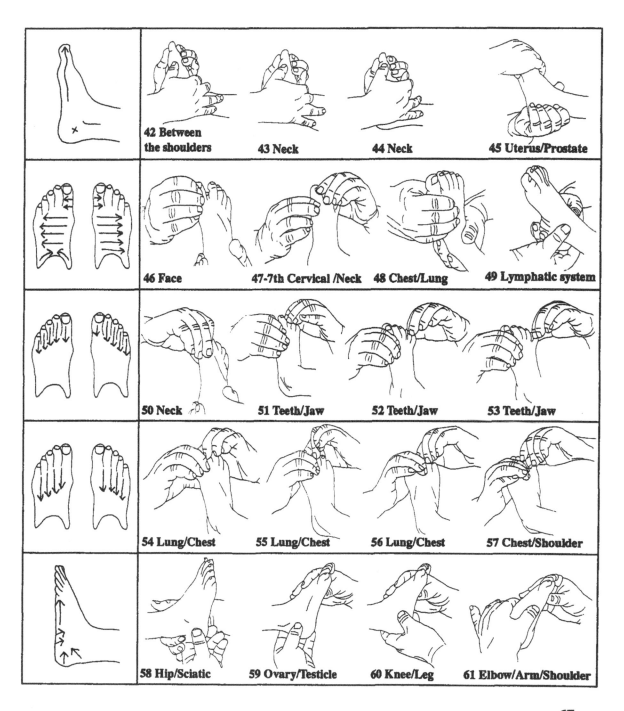

67

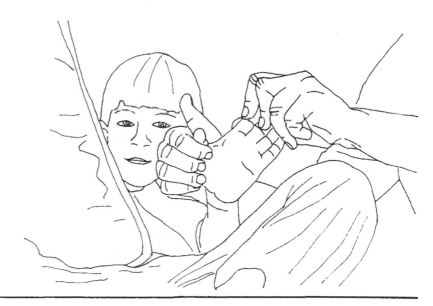

Chapter 4   Hand Reflexology

The hands provide a convenient site for reflexology work. They are easily accessible and, at times, they are the most appropriate location for your work. Jane, for example, picked up her daughter's hand to work in the casualty department. Applying technique to a foot would not have been appropriate. If the foot or ankle is injured, the hand is chosen for work. When working with a chronic condition, such as hay fever, the hands provide ready access for the amount of work needed.

The hands reflect stresses in other parts of the body. While demonstrating at a convention, we were approached by a wife concerned about her husband's chronic habit of cracking his fingers. Indeed, the joints of his fingers were enlarged for a young man. Interestingly enough, he had begun this habit as a child. Years later he had been diagnosed with a scoliosis of the spine. The unconscious habit may have been an attempt to relieve the stress he had always felt in his neck. (As you will see, the fingers reflect the head and neck areas of the body.)

Which is more effective— foot reflexology or hand reflexology? This question is a matter of debate within the reflexology community. In general, the feet are seen to be more responsive to reflexology work. The feet are protected by shoes and thus are more sensitive to touch. The hands have no such protection and are not as sensitive generally. Both have unique advantages, and results can be produced by working with either.

In this chapter, you will learn how to apply hand reflexology techniques, how to read a hand reflexology chart, and how to apply a whole hand workout.

Techniques

To experiment with hand reflexology techniques applied to your own hands, try the exercise outlined in the Foot Reflexology chapter. As you will have noticed, the hands and feet have their own distinctive shapes. The role of the feet is to bear our weight and make walking possible. The role of the hands is to carry weight and manipulate objects.

To consider the effects of reflexology work on the hands, try working with your own hand. Grasp the index finger of the left hand as shown. Now, pull gently, stretching the finger. Hold for fifteen seconds. Try this with each finger of your left hand. Now flex the fingers of both hands. Does the left hand feel differently from the right?

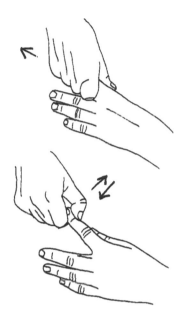

Try another technique. Grasp the joint of the index finger as shown. Now, gently move the finger back and forth, creating sidewise movement at the joint. Try this with each finger of your left hand. Flex the fingers of both hands. How does the feeling of the two hands compare?

As you work with the hands of others, be aware of the effect of your work. Be sensitive to the child's comfort zone. Work on another's hands as you would like them to work on yours.

Quick and easy techniques

Now that you have tried applying pressure techniques to your hands, try it on another. Remember: Begin reflexology work with a light touch. Do not press to your full capacity of strength, and experiment with different strengths of pressure as you explore the techniques.

Single finger grip

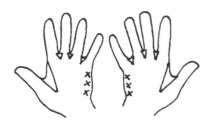

Seat yourself next to your volunteer. Sit to his or her left to apply techniques to the left hand. Rest your hand and the volunteer's hand on a pillow. Place his or her hand in the palm of your hand. Resting the fingertip of your index finger on the palm of the hand, gently press several times. Does this prompt a reaction from the child? Is it painful? Does it tickle? Is it overly strong pressure? (Avoid digging your fingernail into the skin.) Then try this technique in the center of the thumb.

Next, try applying this technique in the webbing of the hand. Rest the thumb and index fingertips on the top and palm surface, respectively. Press the thumb and fingertips together several times. Experiment by moving your fingers to another place in the webbing and pressing. Does the webbing under your fingertips feel differently in different locations? Try this technique with the webbing between the fingers. Does each of the three areas feel differently?

Try this technique with the fleshy outer edge of the hand.

Now try this technique at a joint of a finger. Rather than pressing several times, maintain a steady pressure for a few seconds. Direct pressure such as this creates a pain-killing effect.

Multiple finger grip

The multiple finger grip technique provides pressure to a broader surface of the hand. Rest your fingertips on the palm surface of the hand, as shown. Press with multiple fingertips gently. Experiment with differing levels of pressure. Avoid digging your fingernails into the skin.

Experiment with different parts of the hand.

Grip Technique

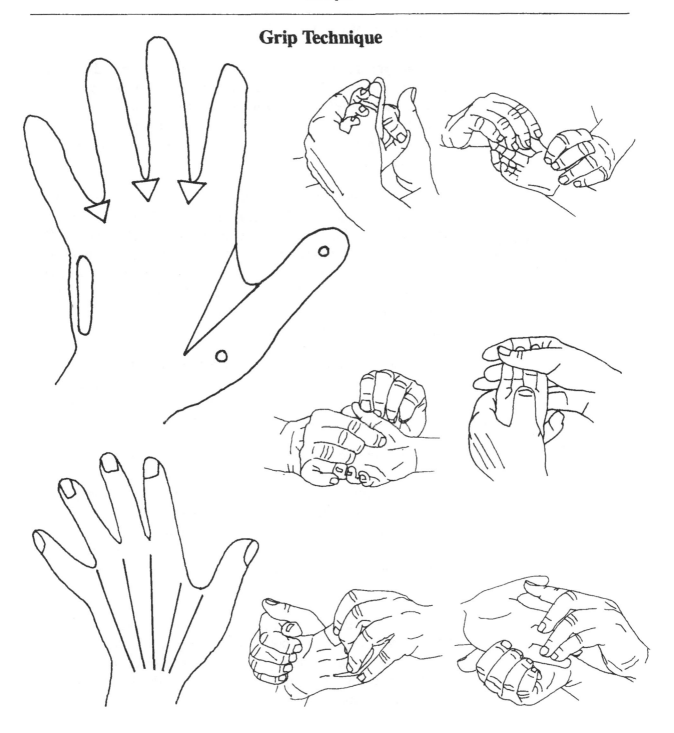

Thumb walking technique

As you have noticed by now, the hand is not the same shape as the foot. This is all the more apparent when applying thumb walking technique to the hand. It takes time to become accustomed to each shape. In general, one hand holds and controls the fingers while the other hand applies thumb walking technique.

To practice using the thumb walking technique on the hand, seat yourself on the right hand side of your volunteer. Rest his or her hand on a pillow, palm side up. With your left hand, stretch the fingers back so that the palm of the hand is open. Rest the fingers of the right hand on the top side of the hand. Place your thumb at the base of the index finger. Now apply the thumb walking technique to the finger. Proceed in the same manner with each finger.

Now try the thumb walking technique in the palm of the hand. Rest the working thumb as shown. Apply the thumb walking technique between the bones. Feel the surface under your thumb. Does it vary? Does the child respond?

Try applying thumb walking technique to other parts of the palm. Rest the working thumb at the base of the child's wrist. The fingers rest on top of the hand for leverage. Apply the thumb walking technique, moving the thumb in a forward direction. Make several passes through the same area. Reposition your thumb at the wrist. Apply the thumb walking technique to another area of the palm. Do you feel differences in the surface under your thumb?

The top of the hand is a bony surface. The troughs between bones form convenient working paths for your thumb walking technique Rest your working thumb at the base of the fingers. Apply the thumb walking technique along the bony trough. Avoid making contact with your fingernails.

Thumb Walking Technique

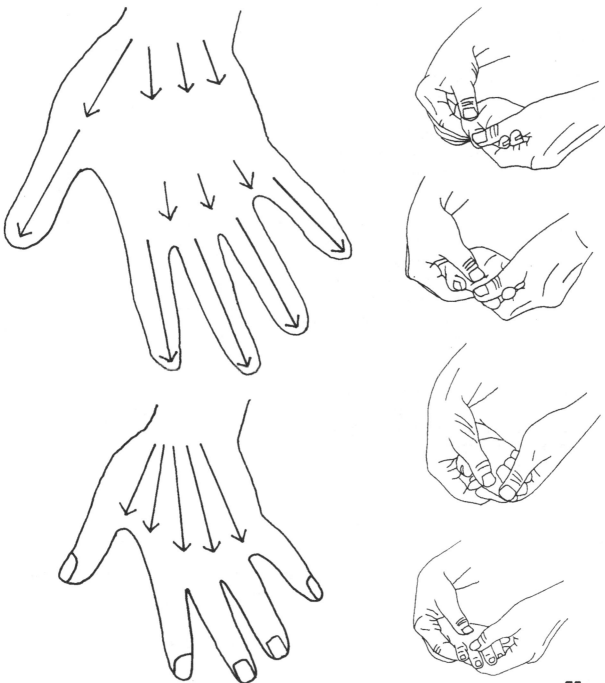

Charts and How to Use Them

Zone Charts

The zones of the hands are ten in number and correspond to each finger and the thumbs. Zones are utilized in reflexology to link the body and hand. Lateral zones provide the ability to further focus efforts. The lateral markers are (A) the base of the neck, (B) the diaphragm, (C) the waistline, and (D) the base of the pelvis.

To practice this, consider a pain in the body. At the time Jane was sitting in the casualty department with her daughter without a medical diagnosis, she used a few charting directions to find a place on her daughter's hand. She then applied technique — a constant, steady pressure for easing the pain. Jane knew her daughter's pain was on the right side and below the waistline.

Note the location of "X" in the illustration of the body. Note that "X" lies on the right side of the body. Note that the "X" lies in zone 5 of the body. To find the zone as represented on the hand, consider zone 5 of the right hand. Note the marker of the "Waistline."

Notice that the thumb includes five zones. The thumb thus represents half of the head area as well as one specific zone.

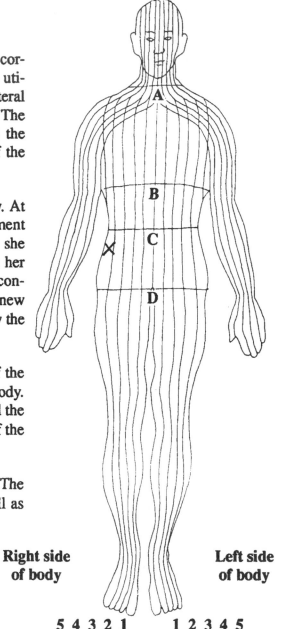

**Right side
of body**

**Left side
of body**

5 4 3 2 1   1 2 3 4 5

Zone Charts

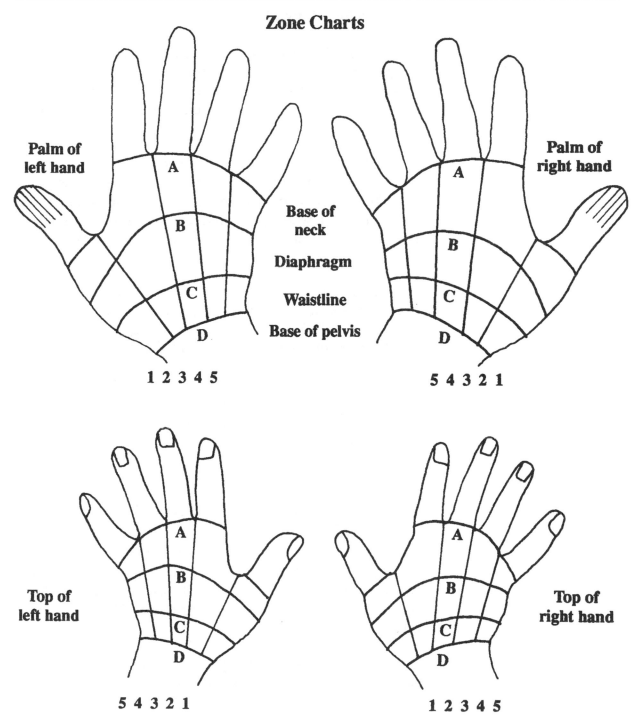

Palm of
left hand

Palm of
right hand

Base of
neck

Diaphragm

Waistline

Base of pelvis

1 2 3 4 5

5 4 3 2 1

Top of
left hand

Top of
right hand

5 4 3 2 1

1 2 3 4 5

Hand reflexology chart

The hand reflexology chart reflects a mirror image of the body on the hand. It is a map of the organs within the gridlike zone system. It is used as a specific tool to focus on specific organs, systems, or functions of the body that may be under stress.

For example, a woman considered leaving a lecture we were giving because of stomach upset. During the course of the talk, she had followed the example we were demonstrating and applied pressure with a golf ball (see next page) to her stomach area. She stayed until the end of the lecture because of the technique's effectiveness.

As you can see, use of the reflexology chart in this manner is a fast and simple way to locate and work with areas of concern. The simple formula of "finding a sore spot and rubbing it out" has been successful for many individuals.

There are further strategies for reflexology technique application. For specific strategies, see the chapters "Workouts" and "Conditions." The ideal situation for technique application is work over the hand as a whole.

The Whole Hand Workout

Technique applied to the whole hand provides several benefits. One is relaxation from stress for growing hands. Young hands learning to write or spending hours over computer keyboards need the relaxation from their efforts. Hand injury is a very real fact of life.

The whole hand workout gives you an opportunity to compare and contrast the "feel" of one part of the hand to another. Over time especially this thorough workout can give you a

Hand Reflexology Chart

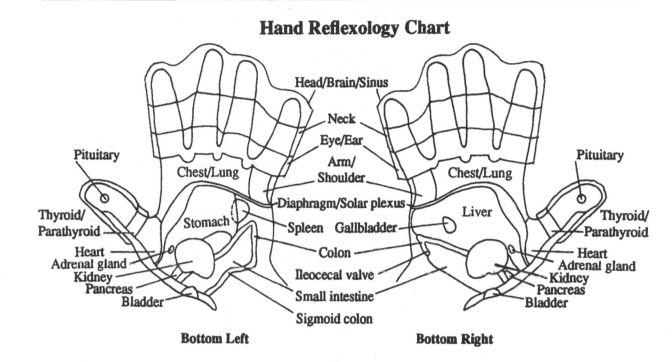

Head/Brain/Sinus
Neck
Eye/Ear
Arm/ Shoulder
Diaphragm/Solar plexus
Spleen   Gallbladder
Colon
Ileocecal valve
Small intestine
Sigmoid colon

Pituitary
Thyroid/ Parathyroid
Heart
Adrenal gland
Kidney
Pancreas
Bladder
Chest/Lung
Stomach

Liver
Chest/Lung
Pituitary
Thyroid/ Parathyroid
Heart
Adrenal gland
Kidney
Pancreas
Bladder

Bottom Left   **Bottom Right**

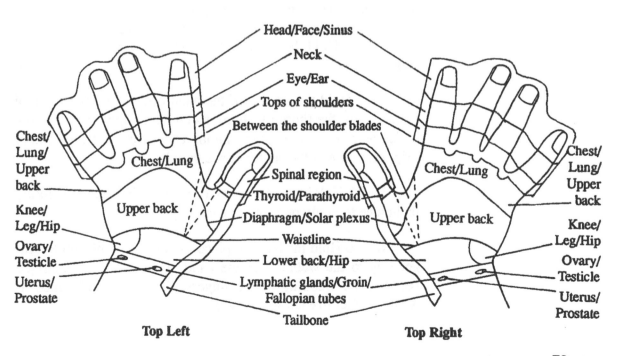

Head/Face/Sinus
Neck
Eye/Ear
Tops of shoulders
Between the shoulder blades
Spinal region
Thyroid/Parathyroid
Diaphragm/Solar plexus
Waistline
Lower back/Hip
Lymphatic glands/Groin/ Fallopian tubes
Tailbone

Chest/ Lung/ Upper back
Knee/ Leg/Hip
Ovary/ Testicle
Uterus/ Prostate
Chest/Lung
Upper back

Chest/Lung
Upper back
Chest/ Lung/ Upper back
Knee/ Leg/Hip
Ovary/ Testicle
Uterus/ Prostate

Top Left   **Top Right**

79

broader frame of reference for your reflexology work. You will be familiar with the feel of the child's hand and can tell that a change in stress level has occurred. You will develop the ability to feel that change has occurred in response to your work.

Finally, the whole hand is provided with exercise. Since relaxation is the basic goal within reflexology's philosophy, a whole hand workout is more effective in reaching this goal. Also, working with the entire hand provides a more holistic approach in general.

Work on the right hand is illustrated. A full workout would include work on both hands. Illustrations are given of the reflex areas of the left hand which are not common to both hands.

1 Begin your workout by checking to see if there are any areas to be aware of, such as cuts or bruises. Avoid work on these areas. Cover with a bandage to avoid working.

2–6 Begin your work with a series of dessert/relaxation techniques, the finger pull. Grasp the finger with the working hand and the wrist with the holding hand. Gently pull the finger toward you. Hold the position for a few seconds. Go on to each finger.

7–10 Hold the fingers of the hand back with your holding hand. Using the thumb walking technique, apply pressure in a series of passes across the thumb. Then use the single finger grip technique in the center of the thumb.

11–14 Holding the fingers back, use the thumb walking technique to apply pressure to each finger.

15 –18 Hold the hand in place as you apply the single Finger grip to the webbing of the hand. Then, use the technique between the webbing of the fingers. (Is there a difference in what you feel in each webbing?)

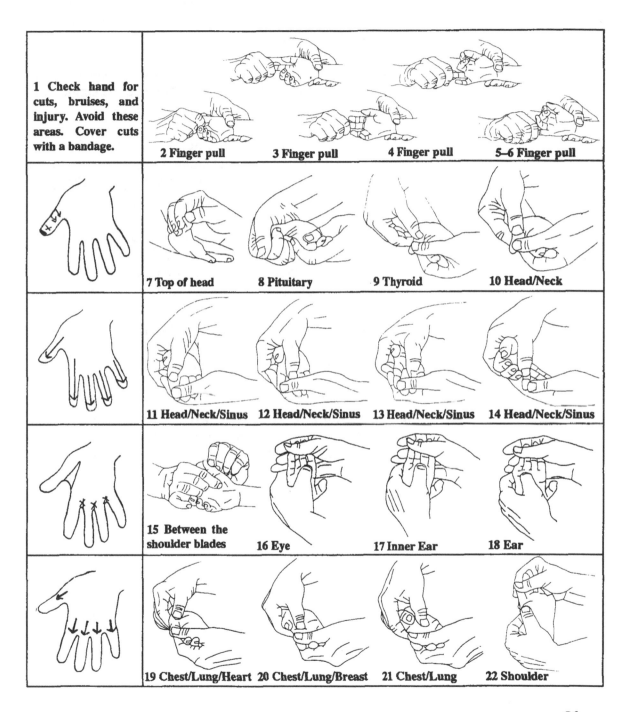

1 Check hand for cuts, bruises, and injury. Avoid these areas. Cover cuts with a bandage.

2 Finger pull   3 Finger pull   4 Finger pull   5–6 Finger pull

7 Top of head   8 Pituitary   9 Thyroid   10 Head/Neck

11 Head/Neck/Sinus   12 Head/Neck/Sinus   13 Head/Neck/Sinus   14 Head/Neck/Sinus

15 Between the shoulder blades   16 Eye   17 Inner Ear   18 Ear

19 Chest/Lung/Heart   20 Chest/Lung/Breast   21 Chest/Lung   22 Shoulder

81

19–22 Hold the fingers of the hand in a stretched position. Apply the thumb walking technique. Make a series of successive passes through the area.

23–26 Hold the fingers of the hand in a stretched position. Apply the thumb walking technique. Then use the single finger grip technique to pinpoint the center of the area.

27–30 Continue to hold the fingers in a stretched position. Apply the thumb walking technique in a series of passes through the area. Then use the single finger grip technique to apply pressure to the fatty outer edge of the hand.

31–35 Hold the hand in a stationary position. Apply the thumb walking technique to the heel of the hand. Then apply thumb walking technique across the area. Now use the single finger grip technique to pinpoint the two deep areas indicated.

36–38 Hold the hand in a stationary position so that the thumb side is turned toward you. Apply the thumb walking technique in a series of successive passes.

39–43 Apply the finger pull technique. Grasp the finger with the working hand and the wrist with the holding hand. Gently pull the finger toward you. Hold the position for a few seconds. Go on to each finger.

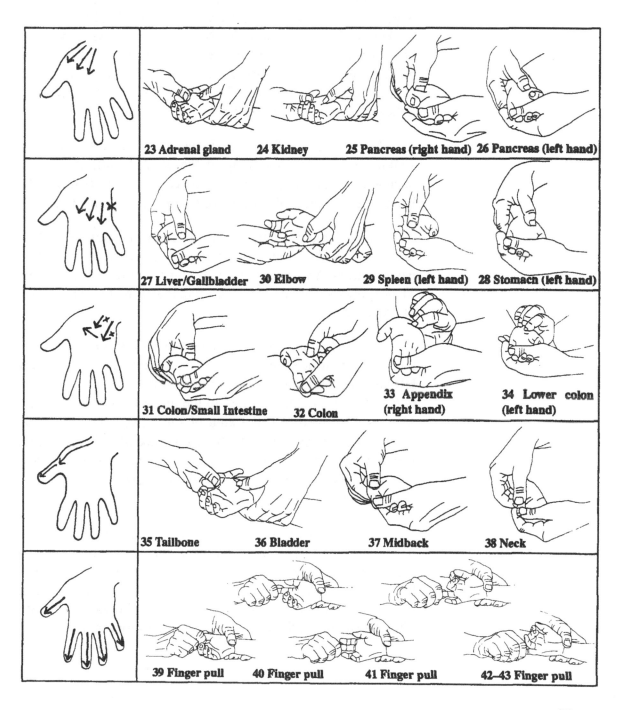

23 Adrenal gland   24 Kidney   25 Pancreas (right hand) 26 Pancreas (left hand)

27 Liver/Gallbladder 30 Elbow   29 Spleen (left hand) 28 Stomach (left hand)

31 Colon/Small Intestine   32 Colon   33 Appendix (right hand)   34 Lower colon (left hand)

35 Tailbone   36 Bladder   37 Midback   38 Neck

39 Finger pull 40 Finger pull 41 Finger pull 42–43 Finger pull

44–47 Turn the hand so that the top is available for your work. Hold the hand in a steady position. Apply the finger walking technique to the wrist. Make several passes covering a broad area. Then pinpoint the deep area of the hand indicated. With the holding hand turn the child's hand in a circle. An on-off pressure is thus created. Now pinpoint the other deep area indicated and move the child's hand in a circle.

48–51 Hold the fingers and steady the hand. Apply thumb walking technique, beginning at the wrist. Continue to apply technique in the trough formed between the long bones of the hand. Make a series of successive passes through the area.

52–55 Hold the hand to steady it. Apply thumb walking technique to the index finger. Make a series of successive passes across the finger, with particular attention to the joints. Then apply the technique to each finger and the thumb in a similar manner.

56–58 Hold the hand with your left hand to steady it. Place the fingertip in one area indicated by a circle. Now, with your left holding hand move the hand in the direction of a circle. An on/off pressure is thus applied to the area under your fingertip. Move your fingertip to the area of the wrist indicated by the other circle. Repeat the described procedure. Apply thumb walking technique in the direction indicated by the arrows of the illustration. Make several successive passes creating a thorough coverage.

59–63 Grasp the index finger. Each of your hands holds the finger at a joint. The hand grasping the lower joint remains motionless, holding the finger in a fixed position. The fingers of the other hand move the finger at the upper joint from side to side. Then apply technique to each finger and the thumb. Note: This is a small, gentle movement. Do not apply force.

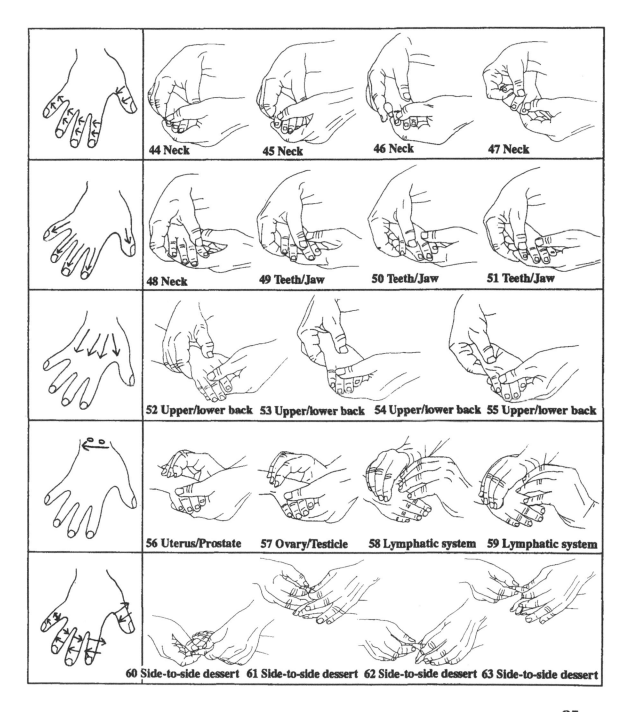

44 Neck   45 Neck   46 Neck   47 Neck

48 Neck   49 Teeth/Jaw   50 Teeth/Jaw   51 Teeth/Jaw

52 Upper/lower back   53 Upper/lower back   54 Upper/lower back   55 Upper/lower back

56 Uterus/Prostate   57 Ovary/Testicle   58 Lymphatic system   59 Lymphatic system

60 Side-to-side dessert   61 Side-to-side dessert   62 Side-to-side dessert   63 Side-to-side dessert

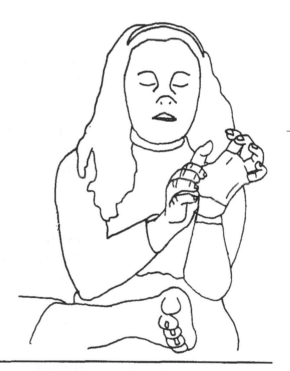

Chapter 5 Workouts

Within the traditions of reflexology, patterns of technique application have been developed to most efficiently and effectively create results. The pattern consists of technique application, a target or targets, and the timing of efforts. These "ingredients" combine to create the right experience for you and your child. Your investment of time and effort will be enhanced by using the technique pattern that is tailored to your child's needs.

The reflexology workouts in this chapter have been created to enable you to best focus your efforts. Just as with self-improvement through exercise, success in applying reflexology results from a focused effort. The more specific your goal, the more specific your work. For example, when Jane sought to ease her daughter's pain, she applied a specific workout that was different from the one she used when her daughter injured an ankle playing soccer.

The following workouts have the potential to give you and your child successful results using reflexology. Achieving results will, we hope, lead on to your further exploration and success. Remember, Jane succeeded because she tried.

Reaching Your Goal with a Reflexology Workout

To simplify the traditional patterns of technique application, we have created ten workouts that will most effectively help you to meet your goals. Those who succeed using this approach have discovered the right ingredients:

•Locating target areas: Where to apply pressure

•Applying pressure: How much pressure to apply and for how long

•Reading feedback: How to assess technique application

Locating target areas

The building blocks for the workouts that follow in this chapter are the target areas for technique application: mirror image areas, specific reflex areas, mirror function areas and helper areas.

Mirror image area

As noted in Chapter 3, the image of the body is mirrored on the feet and hands. To locate a target area on the feet or hands, consider the relationship between the feet or hands and the body. The markers signifying the relationship are the base of the neck, diaphragm, waistline, and base of the pelvis.

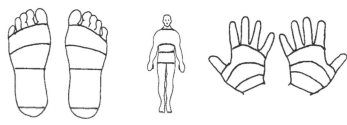

Specific reflex areas

Many people have successfully applied reflexology using these specific reflex areas. As you have seen with the reflexology chart and as you will see in Chapter 6, reflexology theory includes the use of a one-or two-step approach. Pressure technique is applied to one or two areas of the foot or hand to achieve results.

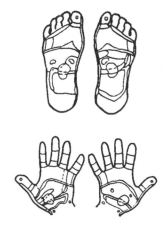

Mirror function area

As noted in Chapter 3, pressure technique is also applied to influence a function of the body. To use reflexology technique to influence a function, see Chapter 6 and note the descriptions of anatomical function listed with each body part.

Helper areas

At times, better results can be achieved by working with helper areas. The helper areas include the reflex areas of the systems of the body; for example, the stomach as a part of the digestive system. Referral areas relate one limb of the body to another. Zones relate one part of the body to another.

Systems of the body

In response to stress, a system of the body responds as a whole to provide fuel and locomotive capability. In choosing which areas of the foot you will apply technique application emphasis, consider the reflex areas of the entire system. For example, if the reflex area of a particular organ shows sensitivity on the hand or foot, find out whether there is the sensitivity in the reflex areas of other organs within that system. For further information, see Chapter 6.

Endocrine system: Pituitary, adrenal glands, pancreas, ovary/testicle, uterus/prostate

Digestive system: Stomach, gallbladder, liver, pancreas, small intestine, large intestine

Urinary system: Kidneys, ureter tubes, bladder

Reproductive system: Ovary, uterus, fallopian tubes (for females); testicles, prostate (for males)

Nervous system: Spinal cord, brain

Cardiovascular system: Heart, arteries, veins

Lymphatic system: Lymph ducts, spleen, thymus

Immune system: Liver, spleen, endocrine system, lymphatic system

Respiratory system: Lungs

Referral Areas

At times, better results are achieved if pressure is applied to "referral areas." Within reflexology theory, referral areas are those areas where you would apply pressure if you are not able to apply pressure to the specific reflex area because of the injury there or as helper areas to the specific reflex areas. For example, when Jane's daughter injured her ankle, we showed her self-help techniques to apply to a referral area on her hand.

The referral areas relate the toes to fingers, foot to hand, calf to forearm, knee to elbow, thigh to upper arm and hip to shoulder.

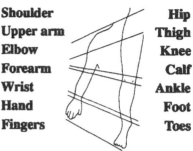

Shoulder	Hip
Upper arm	Thigh
Elbow	Knee
Forearm	Calf
Wrist	Ankle
Hand	Foot
Fingers	Toes

Referral areas

Zones

At times, better results are achieved if pressure is applied along the entire zone of the foot or hand. The feet and hands have been found to be particularly effective in providing a location for such influence. To influence a body part, one applies pressure anywhere along the zone. The body part is thus influenced by applying pressure to the appropriate zone of the foot or hand.

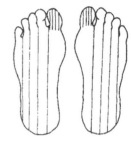

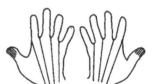

Applying pressure

Any time pressure is applied to the feet or hands, the body reacts. Just as Goldilocks was looking for porridge that was just the right temperature at the three bears' house, you are seeking just the right ingredients to most effectively and efficiently get results.

How much pressure to apply, how long to apply pressure, and how frequently to apply pressure will vary from situation to situation. The child who was using the golf ball to help with his migraine headaches, for example, had evidently found the right formula — he knew how much pressure and how long to continue to apply it to get results.

Challenge level

To find the right formula, you will want to match your reflexology technique application to a challenge level appropriate to the child's situation. Three types of situations generally arise and become the goal for reflexology technique application.

One goal is to use reflexology to interrupt a current situation, such as an injury, pain, an allergy or asthma attack, stress, or cold symptoms.

Another goal is to apply reflexology in a circumstance where a condition has become chronic over time. Situations include a past injury, an on-going illness, or prolonged stress.

A third goal of reflexology technique application is to bolster the body's natural efforts towards health with preventive application.

In each of the workouts, you will see that as circumstances change, you will change the workout. What you will be adjusting is your targeted areas, the amount of pressure you exert, how frequently you apply technique, and over what time period you apply technique.

Both you and your child will become adept at changing techniques to achieve the results you are seeking. As your work progresses, continually consider the effects of your work. What exactly do you consider a benefit of your work? As one client commented, "I suddenly realized I could turn my head when driving to look at the traffic behind me." Effects can be subtle. With a child, the best gauge may be his or her mood. Has it improved? Is he or she sleeping better? What other indicators of change can you see?

Appropriate use of reflexology

An important part of reflexology theory is deciding when to use reflexology and when not to use it. Do not use reflexology techniques to work directly on:

- a cut
- a bruise
- an injured hand or foot, wrist or ankle
- any part of the foot or hand that is injured
- an ingrown nail
- corns
- a rash
- plantar wart
- split skin between toes
- athlete's foot
- callousing that is cracked
- any foot problem that requires the attention of a chiropodist

Do not diagnose with reflexology. There is a difference between a diagnosis and an assessment. One can make an assessment of stress using reflexology. Never use reflexology to diagnose critical issues involving your child's health. Reflexology provides input, but it should not constitute the basis for your actions. Follow standard first aid or a medically recommended response first.

Do not work on a reflex area that is overly sensitive. Do not overwork a part of the foot or hand. For instance, an infection in the body will be reflected as a very sensitive area on the foot or hand. If you are working on yourself, it is at that point where the foot or hand feels tender or bruised to the touch. Working on others, it is more difficult to judge this, especially with very young children, who have no words to express themselves. Pulling the foot away and breaking into tears are signs of overstress.

Reading feedback

As you apply reflexology techniques, you will probably notice two things: one, your work creates a response from the child, and two, what you feel under your thumb will vary from area to area. The child's response and what you feel provide information to assess your reflexology work. By considering such things, you can get a feel for the child's level of stress.

Sensitivity

One of the simplest ways to assess a child's feet is through sensitivity to technique application. An area that is sensitive is usually under some form of stress. A response of "Ouch" from her son when she pressed the stomach reflex area helped one mother determine whether or not her son was faking a stomach ache to avoid going to school.

A child who removes a foot or hand from your grasp as a result of technique application is definitely showing sensitivity. Rather than fighting through a wall of pain, consider alternate areas for your work.

Nonverbal communication

It is a basic tenet of reflexology that pressing on the foot or hand will cause an effect throughout the body. It is also true, however, that in applying reflexology technique to the foot or hand, you are applying pressure to a foot or hand. As any professional reflexologist will tell you, the person you are working on will react to your technique application. With children, that reaction is a bit more complicated. As noted above, the child will respond by indicating sensitivity. In addition, nonverbal communication is all important with children.

Young children often do not have the words to express their reactions to your work. Also, children do not have the same response to pressure application that adults do. While an adult will respond with an expression of pain, a child will squirm as if to escape. (Some may leave at this point if you do not quickly soften your approach. They are harsh critics.) When asked, "Does that hurt," they will say, "No, it feels funny" or "No, it tickles." At this point, you should always ask, "Do you want me to go on?" Children will almost always say yes.

The reaction of an older child will more closely parallel that of an adult. In answer to the question "Does that hurt?" they may say something like, "Yes, but it hurts good" or "No, it hurts bad" Your next question should be "Do you want me to go on?" When you proceed, you will should proceed with respect for the newly identified sore area.

Developing a sense of feel

As you work on your child's feet or hands, you will gain more and more of a sense of feel. The pattern of stress you feel under your thumb will create target areas for technique application. You will notice the change in the feel as your work progresses or as stress factors enter your child's life.

The reflex areas have characteristics on which technique application should be further evaluated. As you work with the feet or hands of the child, consider what you feel under your thumb. If your child has experienced chronic asthma, for example, consider the feel of the appropriate areas on the hands or feet. Now try the same thing with a child who does not experience chronic asthma and you will see the difference.

Workouts

Interrupting the stress of the moment

A current stress is one that is happening right now. A recent injury or a current illness or an emotional stress calls for a particular strategy. It calls for gently applied technique to specific targeted parts of the foot or hand during the stress period. The following workouts describe successful strategies you can use to interrupt the stress of the moment.

Workout: To help recovery process

One-year-old Amanda chose to take her first steps in the out-of-doors. Her parents watched in horror as she walked and fell — right into a campfire. Her hands and face were burned, with a possibility of scarring and an impaired use of the hand. As her mother rocked her and carried her while she was recuperating in the hospital, a few gentle squeezes were effectively applied as a part of her comforting efforts.

The palms of both hands had experienced third-degree burns, with a potential for tendon damage. The application of technique was to the part of the foot corresponding to the hand, virtually the sole of the foot. Pressure was easily applied to the small foot of the one-year-old.

A gentle approach was called for because the child's tension level was heightened due to the injury. Any strong application of technique might be counterproductive, by providing too much challenge. Working with the whole foot or hand spreads out the challenge of technique. Applying technique every fifteen minutes creates a frequency of pattern.

Workout: To help the recovery process		
Consider a goal	**Step 1: Set goal**	• Influence a current injury • Influence the chronic effects of injury
Choose where to work	**Step 2: Locate target area (choose one)**	• Locate mirror image • Locate specific reflex area of hand or foot. • Locate referral area • Locate zone • CAUTION: Do not work directly on an injured area.
Choose when to work	**Step 3: Apply pressure (choose one)**	Current: • Generalized gentle pressing and squeezing of the foot or hand, whichever is easily available. Make contact. Let the body bounce back. Don't add too much challenge at this stage. • Be consistent. Be frequent. Every fifteen minutes of a soft press to a specific area is not too much.
		Chronic effects of injury: • Apply pressure while observing the child's reaction to it • Gradually add more target areas (see above list) • Apply a whole foot workout twice a week with emphasis (extra work) on specific areas • Add the injury to your child's health history of stressed areas (see Special Uses) • Show the child some self-help techniques (see Special Uses)
Listen	**Step 4: Feedback**	Watch for: • Results: Did the stress level change? • Sensitivity: Is the area sensitive? • Nonverbal communication: Did the child's body language tell you something? • Sense of feel: What did you feel?
Evaluate	**Step 5**	• Did you get results? • If not, choose another target area and try again.

Workout: Easing pain

As described earlier, Jane utilized a reflexology technique to ease her daughter's pain while they were waiting for medical care. Within reflexology theory, direct pressure applied to a specific part of the foot or hand is utilized to ease pain. The direct pressure is exerted for fifteen to thirty seconds. The specific area has to do with locating the target area of the foot or hand.

Jane located the reflex area corresponding to her daughter's pain because she had a rough idea of the reflex charting of the hand. Her daughter's pain was on the right side of her body, which drew Jane's attention to the right hand. The pain was to the outside of the body and below the waistline. Jane found the "waistline" marker on the hand. She found a sensitive area in the general area she was pressing.

Workout: Easing pain		
Consider a goal	**Step 1: Set goal**	CAUTION: If pain is suddenly urgent and persistent, seek medical help.
Choose where to work	**Step 2: Locate target area (Choose one.)**	• Locate mirror image • Locate specific reflex area of hand or foot • Locate referral area • Locate the zone • CAUTION: Do not work directly on an injured area
Choose when to work	**Step 3: Apply pressure**	Current pain: • Apply direct pressure to a target area for fifteen to thirty seconds to compete with and block the pain signal. • Assess the level of pain. • Reapply direct pressure. Always work within the child's pain tolerance.
		Chronic pain: • Whole foot workout to help the whole body adapt to the stress of pain in one part once or twice a week • Show the child a relevant self-help technique
Listen	**Step 4: Feedback**	Watch for: • Results • Sensitivity • Nonverbal communication • Sense of feel
Evaluate	**Step 5**	• Did you get results? • If not, choose another target area and try again.

Workout: First aid

Standard first aid and medical care are, of course, preferable in any emergency situation. Always call emergency services and administer standard first aid first. There are times and situations, however, when reflexology technique can be applied until help arrives. Reflexology technique has been utilized with first aid situations of revival, shock, and pain.

Reflexology work is **not** appropriate as a primary response. It is not appropriate for use in all situations. Do not work on an injured hand or foot. See referral area. Do not move an injured individual to facilitate your work.

First Aid Workouts	
Goal	**Technique Application**
Revival	Apply pressure to pituitary reflex area. Pump it until results are produced.
Shock	Reduce the potential impact of shock. Use a quiet touch. Provide a calming influence on the body. Just making contact with the foot or hand will calm an agitated child. The solar plexus is a good general calmative area.
Allergic reaction (asthma, hay fever)	Apply pressure to adrenal gland reflex area. Pump it until results are produced.
Anxiety	Apply gentle pressure to solar plexus, adrenal gland, and pancreas reflex areas.
Feedback	Watch for: • Positive result from technique application • Sensitivity • Nonverbal communication • Sense of feel

Workout: Relaxation

Adults who describe childhood reflexology experiences speak in terms of helping the child to feel good and relax. It is difficult to measure the impact of childhood reflexology over a lifetime. Providing a relaxing experience for the child can be very important during times of illness, injury, or stress. Among other things, the child's stress level has been tied to his or her ability to recover from an illness or injury.

The ultimate goal of reflexology is relaxation. To create a relaxing reflexology experience, consider these general guidelines:

Relaxation Workouts	
Workout Strategy	**Technique Application**
Relaxed setting	Arrange the setting. Applying reflexology technique is a matter of timing. Bed time, nap time, or bath time will provide a pleasant association between quiet time and reflexology. Begin with a few soft squeezes.
Relieve stress	Apply gentle pressure technique to the solar plexus reflex area.
Child's favorite areas	Use the child's favorite reflex area or dessert technique. During the course of your work, the child may comment, "That feels good" or "Do that again." Keep these areas in mind for future relaxation use.
Dessert session	Dessert techniques both soothe and distract. The application of technique provides relaxation.
Light touch session	Apply technique concentrating on soothing: Match your technique application to the mood you want to set. A relaxing mood is created by applying a soft touch.
Feedback	Watch for: • Results • Nonverbal communication

Breaking up stress patterns

Health problems, ongoing illness, and chronic injuries form patterns of stress within the body. The role of reflexology is to provide a pattern of pressure techniques to counter the stress pattern. The amount of time needed varies. depending on the pattern of stress.

Techniques vary from goal to goal, but a rule of thumb is
• the longer the condition/injury has existed
• the more the adaptation to stress has taken place
• the more conditioning by technique application will be required
• over a longer period of time
to reach your goal.

Current stress

We were demonstrating at a health show in California when a young woman appeared at the booth. She was experiencing her first painful menstrual period. She sat down in the chair clutching her abdomen. As Barbara worked, applying pressure to the uterus reflex area of the right foot, the young woman gradually sat up straighter and relaxed her hold on her abdomen.

Chronically occurring stress

The reflexology approach to a chronic condition includes applying reflexology technique for an extended period of time. Technique is applied to the specific reflex area, for example, to the adrenal gland reflex area throughout the allergy season, for example, not only during acute attacks.

Prevention

To create a prevention program, technique is applied daily to the specific reflex area. Teaching the child a self-help technique adds to his or her empowerment.

How frequently should the child use the self-help technique? Self-help techniques are rewarding. A positive result from using a self-help technique motivates the child to set his or her schedule according to his or her need. The five-year-old who used a golf ball technique to rid himself of a headache is responding to a problem. But a headache–related allergy might be helped by using the technique on a daily basis.

Health goal workout

The most frequent use of reflexology is to address a specific health concern. Specific parts of the foot or hand are targeted with pressure technique, such as the thumb walking technique or grip, to create a response within the body. The primary targeted area is the reflex area on the foot or hand that mirrors the body part. For example, the bladder reflex area is targeted for bed-wetting.

Another important target is the reflex area that mirrors a body part whose function you want to bolster. For example, the adrenal gland reflex area is targeted in instances where breathing is a concern. One function of the adrenal glands is to produce adrenaline, a hormone used in the treatment of asthma. Another function of the adrenal gland is to fight infection. Thus, for a bladder infection you would target the adrenal reflex area as well as the bladder reflex area.

Reflex areas that mirror systems of the body provide additional areas of interest. Organs, glands, and body parts act together. Organs within one system, for example, affect each other. At times, a whole system can be targeted. For example, the bladder is a part of the urinary system. The kidneys and ureter tubes also play a role in the system. The reflex areas thus also become of interest.

Fighting infections

Children are susceptible to infection as young immune systems learn how to defend themselves. Within reflexology theory, application of technique to the adrenal gland reflex area prompts the infection-fighting responses of the body. So you should work on the adrenal reflex area in addition to working with a specific reflex area when an infection is present.

The stresses of common conditions such as colds, flus, otitis media (middle ear infection), tonsillitis, pneumonia, coxitis (hip joint inflammation), and osteomyelitis may be eased using reflexology techniques in addition to medical help.

Specific reflex areas may sensitize quickly and become too tender for technique application. Consider emphasizing technique application to the adrenal gland reflexes of both hands and feet as well as relevant zones and systems of the body.

Education

For children, the feet are just as important as other parts of a developing body. A workout to meet the goals for improvement would involve a whole foot session twice a week, emphasizing areas. Apply an abbreviated relaxation session at bed time each night to add to a general program of stress reduction and relaxation.

Health Goals Workout		
Consider a goal	Step 1: Set goal	• Influence a current health problem • Influence a chronic health problem • Prevention
Choose where to work	Step 2: Locate target area (choose one)	• Locate relevant mirror image of hand or foot • Locate specific reflex area of hand or foot
Choose when to work	Step 3: Apply pressure	Current health problem: • Apply pressure technique to target area until results are achieved
		Chronic health problem: • Work through the whole foot twice a week with emphasis on specific reflex area • Add reflex areas to work, such as a system related to specific reflex area
		Prevention: • Involve the child in self-help.
Listen	Step 4: Feedback	Watch for: • Results • Sensitivity • Nonverbal communication • Sense of feel
Evaluate	Step 5:	• Did you get results? • If not, choose another target area and try again. • Don't overwork a single reflex area. You've overworked when the reflex area feels sensitive to the touch or bruised. If this occurs, go on to the reflex areas of the system, zone, whole foot, more desserts / general relaxation. When sensitivity has passed, resume your work with the single reflex area. Be aware of the potential for over-work.

Health Concern: Infection		
Concern	Primary Technique Application	Secondary Technique Application
Cold	Apply pressure to adrenal reflex area	Apply pressure to head reflex area (head cold) or lung reflex area (lung cold)
Flu	Apply pressure to adrenal reflex area	Apply pressure to lung reflex area and/or digestive system disorders
Otis media (inner ear infection)	Apply pressure to adrenal reflex area	Apply pressure to inner ear reflex area
Tonsillitis	Apply pressure to adrenal reflex area	Apply pressure to throat reflex area
Pneumonia	Apply pressure to adrenal reflex area	Apply pressure to lung reflex area
Coxitis (hip joint inflammation)	Apply pressure to adrenal reflex area	Apply pressure to hip reflex area
Osteomyelitis (bone marrow inflammation)	Apply pressure to adrenal reflex area	Apply pressure to reflex area corresponding to site of infection

Prevention/Improvement/Development Workouts	
Goal	**Strategy**
Prevention	• Emphasize technique application to areas of the feet or hands that are sensitive to the application
	• Emphasize technique application to endocrine system reflex areas
	• Emphasize technique application to reflex areas relevant to cold, or flu or whatever is going around among children; if it's a sore throat, work the throat reflex area
	• General stress reduction: An overall foot workout, especially at bed time, can help create a deeper level of relaxation
	• Emphasize technique application to reflex areas relevant to something that runs in the family
Improvement	• Emphasize technique application to a system or reflex area
	• Emphasize technique application to endocrine system reflex areas
	• Emphasize technique application to the brain reflex areas
Development	• Emphasize technique application to the reflex areas relevant to a past injury
	• Emphasizing technique application to the endocrine system reflex areas
	• Exercise the foot

Caring

The act of caring in itself is perhaps the greatest contribution of reflexology technique application. Often, simply showing that you care can overcome anything.

At times, it is difficult to know what to do as a parent. A child is sick, injured, or does not seem to be able to verbalize what is bothering him or her — in any number of situations, a parent can be at a loss to know how to proceed in helping the child. Reflexology is a great form of nonverbal communication. It has the ability to reach out and comfort someone when words might not do it.

Do not worry about formality. The goal is to reach out and use touch to establish a physical contact. A frequent response is a general relaxation response or the child may start talking.

Find out what hurts or what is of concern to the child. Has he or she fallen off a bicycle recently? Does a part of the foot hurt sometimes? Apply technique to work toward improvement. The act of working toward a goal of improvement establishes that one cares.

Using reflexology to assess stress

Parents make constant decisions regarding their children's health and well-being. Using reflexology to stay in touch with your child can add to your assessment of a situation. Did Billy hurt his back when he fell today? Should Sally go to school today? While medical attention may not be necessary for either occurrence, nonetheless information provided by the tool of reflexology can contribute to your peace of mind.

Reflexology can be a potential signal for things that may be happening in your child's health. One mother uses it to see whether her child is faking a stomach ache to get out of going to school. (If he says "ouch" when presses the stomach reflex area of his foot is pressed, she knows he is not faking.) Others use reflexology to determine whether the child is under stress that should be attended to. It can serve as an alert that further attention, even medical care, is needed.

1. Note your child's reaction to the work. Is he or she generally sensitive or ticklish? Is he or she sensitive sometimes and not others? Are there times when the child reacts by saying "Ouch" or pulling the foot away?

2. Get to know your child's foot. As you press on the foot, note what you feel under your thumb. You may feel a little lump. To practice noticing such things, press first on the child's foot and then on your own foot or the foot of another. Compare the feet. Do you feel something on one foot and not on another?

3. If your goal is to assess a particular part of the body, select the appropriate reflex area. Apply pressure. What do you feel? Does the child react?

4. Has the child's reaction to your work on the same area changed?

Why results will vary

Exactly what will happen when reflexology's techniques are applied will vary from situation to situation. Specific variables include the individual's age, the individual's general health, and how long a condition has existed.

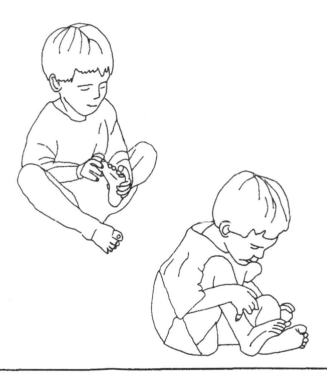

Chapter 6   Conditions/Parts of the Body

Chapter Contents

How to Use This Chapter

This chapter provides information about the reflexology perspective to working with conditions and parts of the body. Where to target and apply pressure is illustrated for a list of common physical conditions and each part of the body.

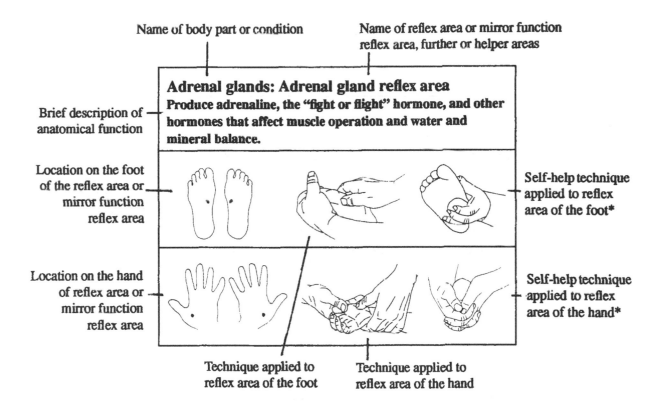

Name of body part or condition

Name of reflex area or mirror function reflex area, further or helper areas

Adrenal glands: Adrenal gland reflex area
Produce adrenaline, the "fight or flight" hormone, and other hormones that affect muscle operation and water and mineral balance.

Brief description of anatomical function

Location on the foot of the reflex area or mirror function reflex area

Self-help technique applied to reflex area of the foot*

Location on the hand of reflex area or mirror function reflex area

Self-help technique applied to reflex area of the hand*

Technique applied to reflex area of the foot

Technique applied to reflex area of the hand

*See page 148. See also Kunz, Kevin and Barbara Kunz, *Hand and Foot Reflexology, A Self-Help Guide*, London, Thorsons, 1984.

Note: A golf ball self-help technique is pictured throughout the chapter. The golf ball technique includes the use of a hard surface applied to soft tissue. Instruct the child to use the golf ball within his or her comfort zone. As noted with the application of other techniques, over-work is possible. A technique application too rigorously applied can create sensitivity.

113

Conditions / Parts of the Body

Adrenal glands: Adrenal gland reflex area
Produce adrenaline, the "fight or flight" hormone, and other hormones that affect muscle operation and water and mineral balance.

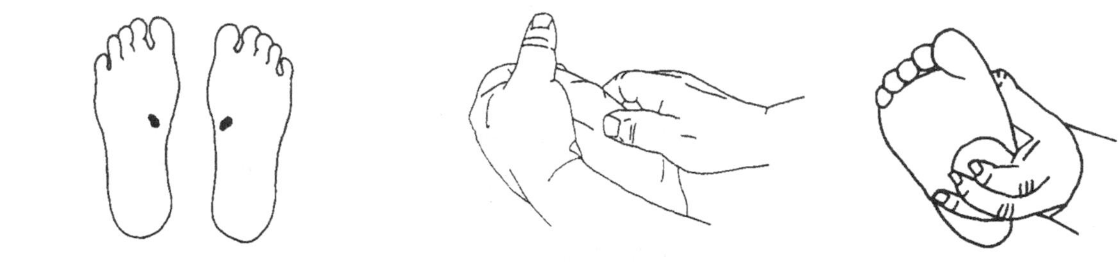

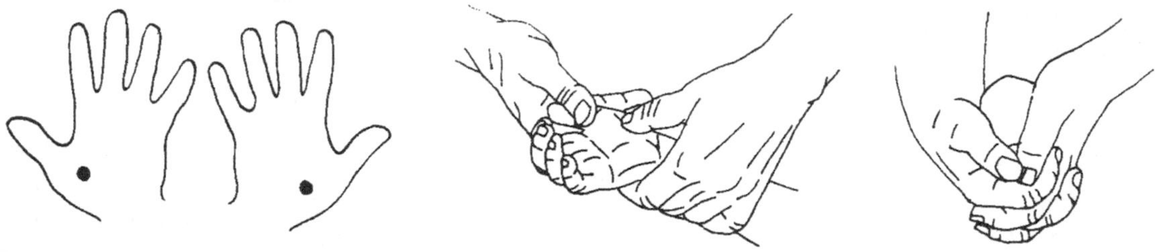

Allergies: Adrenal gland reflex area. *See also* **Lung reflex area.**

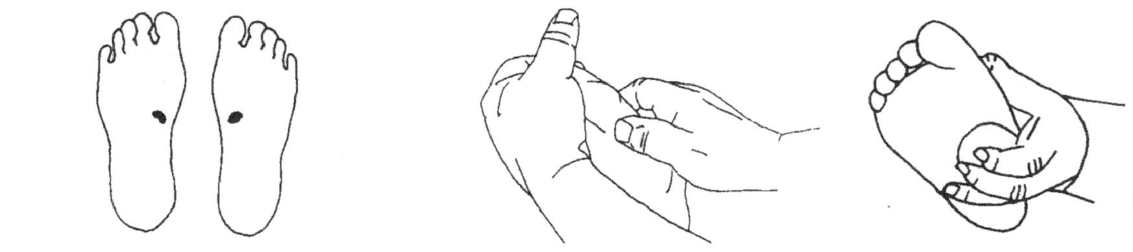

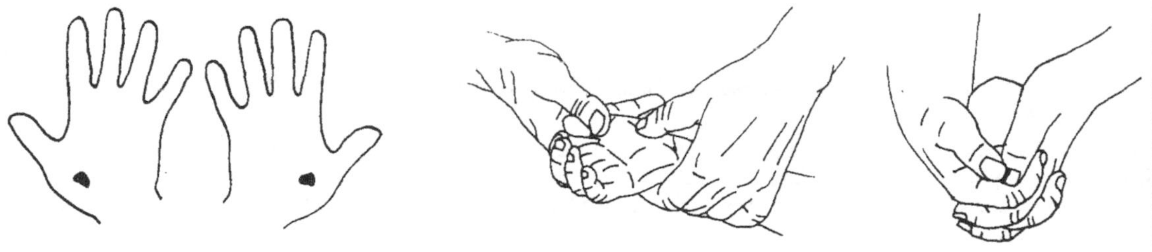

Ankle/Ankle injury: Wrist referral area. CAUTION: Do not work on injured area.

Arm/Arm injury: Arm reflex area. *See also* **Referral areas, p. 91.**

Asthma: Adrenal gland reflex area

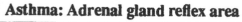
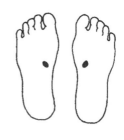
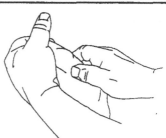
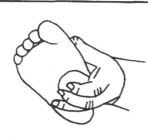

(continued on next page)

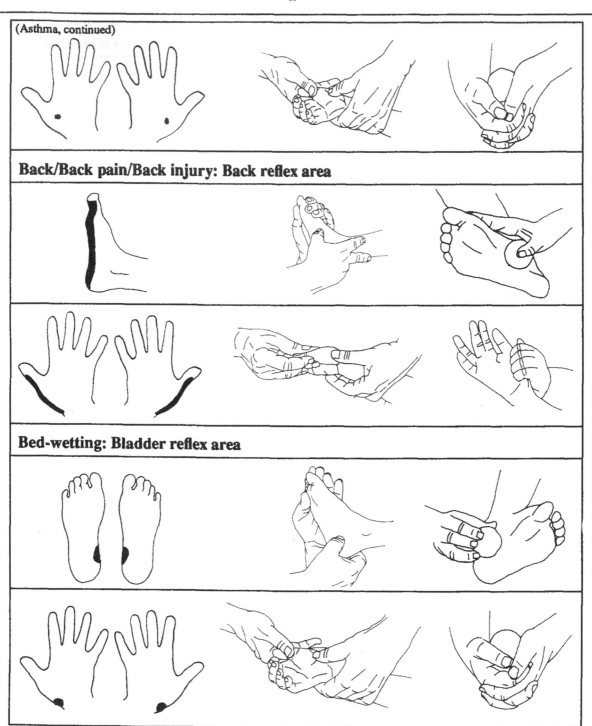

(Asthma, continued)

Back/Back pain/Back injury: Back reflex area

Bed-wetting: Bladder reflex area

Bladder/Bladder infection: Bladder reflex area/Adrenal gland reflex area
Reservoir for urine.

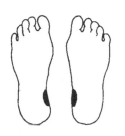 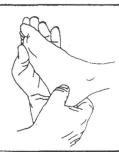 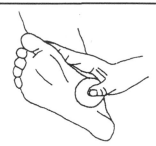

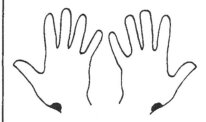 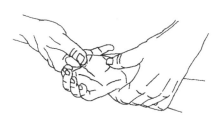 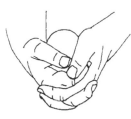

Brain: Brain reflex area
Controls the central nervous system and the endocrine system, which jointly control the whole body. Storage of life's experience and ability to learn.

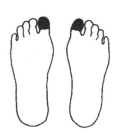 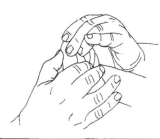 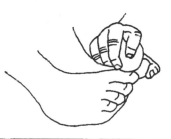

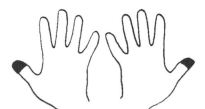 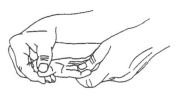 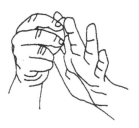

117

Breathing: Adrenal gland reflex area

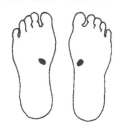 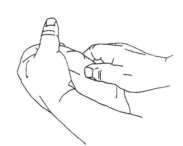 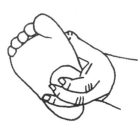

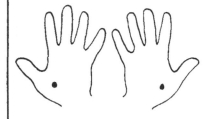 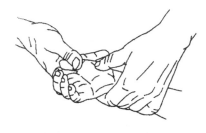 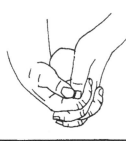

Bronchitis: Lung reflex area/Adrenal gland reflex area

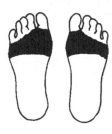 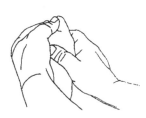 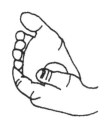

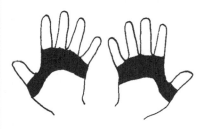 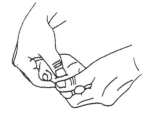 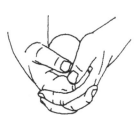

Cardiovascular system: Heart reflex areas
The cardiovascular system is responsible for the constant flow of blood and other body fluids. It consists of the heart, blood vessels, and the lymphatic system.

Heart

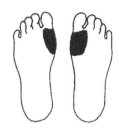

Heart

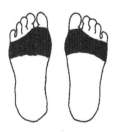 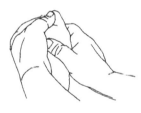 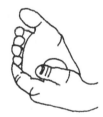

Chest: Chest/Lung/Breast reflex area

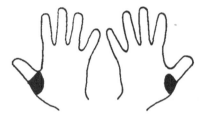

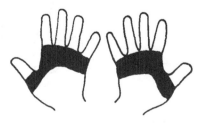 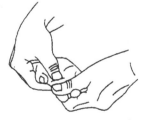 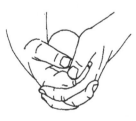

Cold: Head reflex area. *See also* Adrenal gland reflex area.

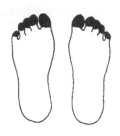 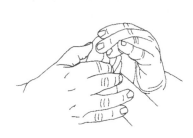 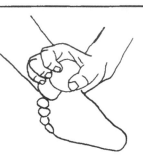

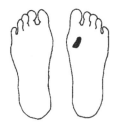 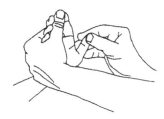 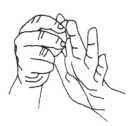

Colic: Digestive system reflex areas

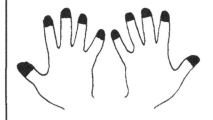 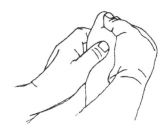 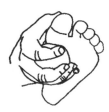

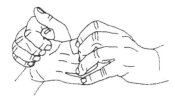 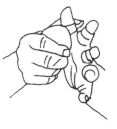

Colon/Small intestine: Colon reflex area. *See also* **Digestive system.**
Absorbs water and electrolytes from waste material. Stores fecal matter.

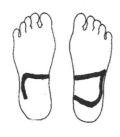 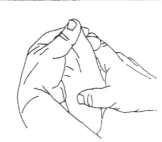 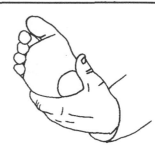

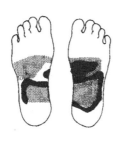 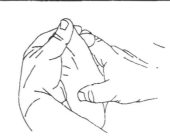 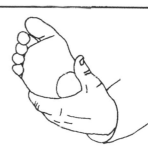

Constipation: Digestive system reflex areas

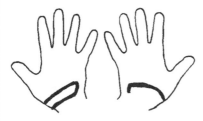 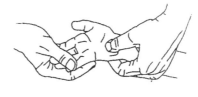 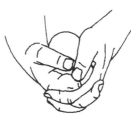

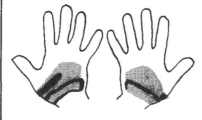 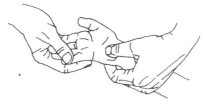 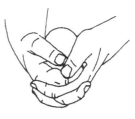

121

Depression: Endocrine system reflex areas

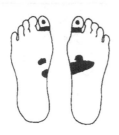 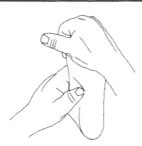 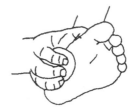

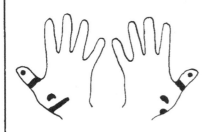 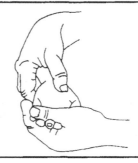 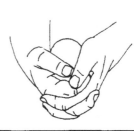

Diabetes: Pancreas reflex area. *See also* Endocrine system.

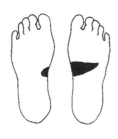 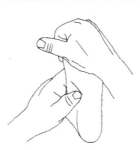 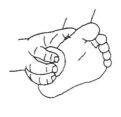

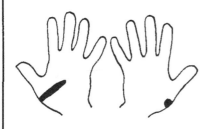 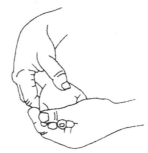 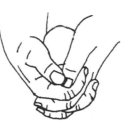

122

Diarrhoea: Digestive system reflex areas

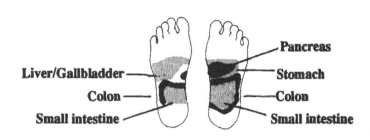

Digestive system: Digestive system reflex areas
The organs of the digestive system are the food processors for the body. Food is ingested, digested, assimilated, then the waste is disposed of. The digestive system includes the stomach, small intestine, colon, liver, and gallbladder.

Pancreas
Stomach
Liver/Gallbladder
Colon
Colon
Small intestine
Small intestine

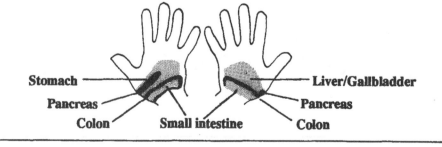

Stomach
Liver/Gallbladder
Pancreas
Pancreas
Colon
Small intestine
Colon

123

Ear/Ear infection: Ear reflex area/Adrenal gland reflex area
Sensory organ which apprises the body of sound.

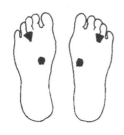 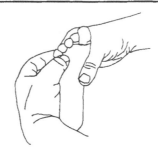 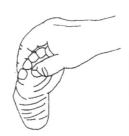

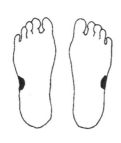 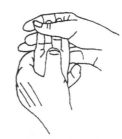 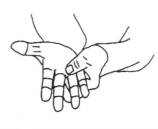

Elbow/Elbow injury: Elbow reflex area. *See also* **Referral areas, p. 91.**

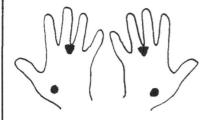 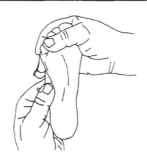 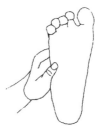

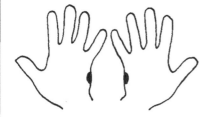 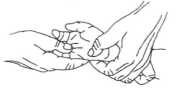 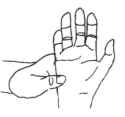

Endocrine system: Endocrine system reflex areas
The endocrine glands are the internal regulators of the body. Through their hormones and with the help of the nervous system, the complex activities of the body are controlled. Vim and vigor, growth and metabolism, and stress and fatigue are all the effects of the endocrine glands.

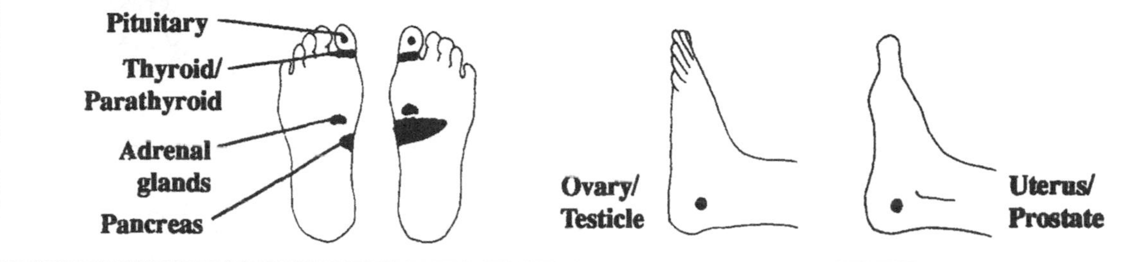

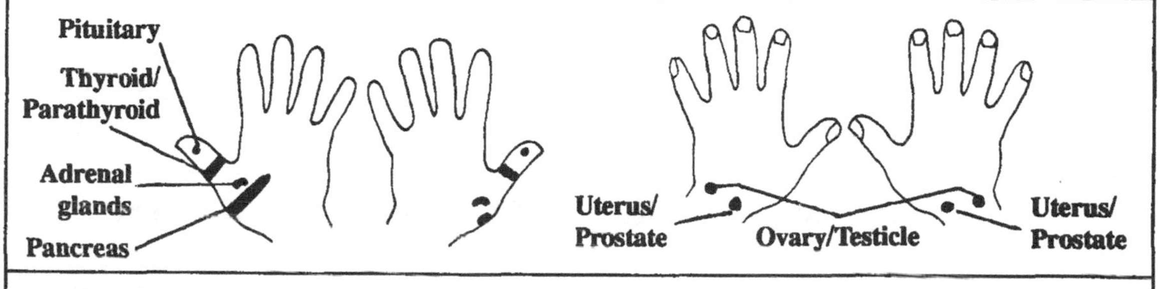

Pituitary
Thyroid/Parathyroid
Adrenal glands
Pancreas

Ovary/Testicle

Uterus/Prostate

Pituitary
Thyroid/Parathyroid
Adrenal glands
Pancreas

Uterus/Prostate

Ovary/Testicle

Uterus/Prostate

Eyes: Eye reflex area
Sensory organ which apprises the body of sight.

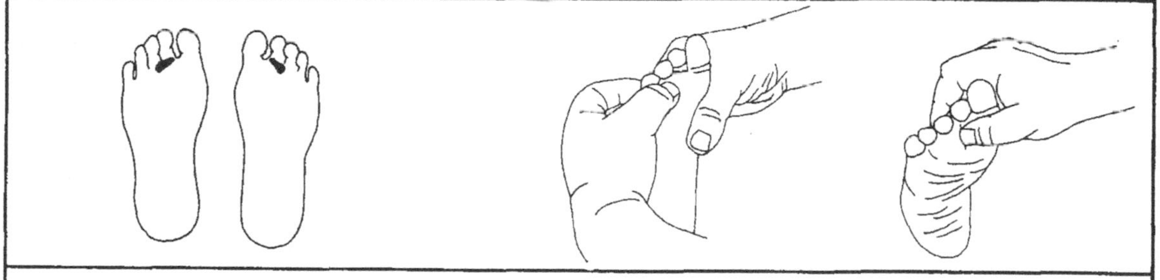

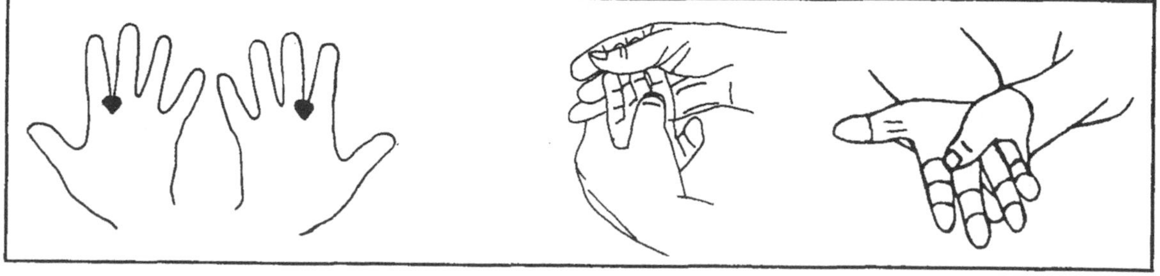

125

Fever: Pituitary reflex area

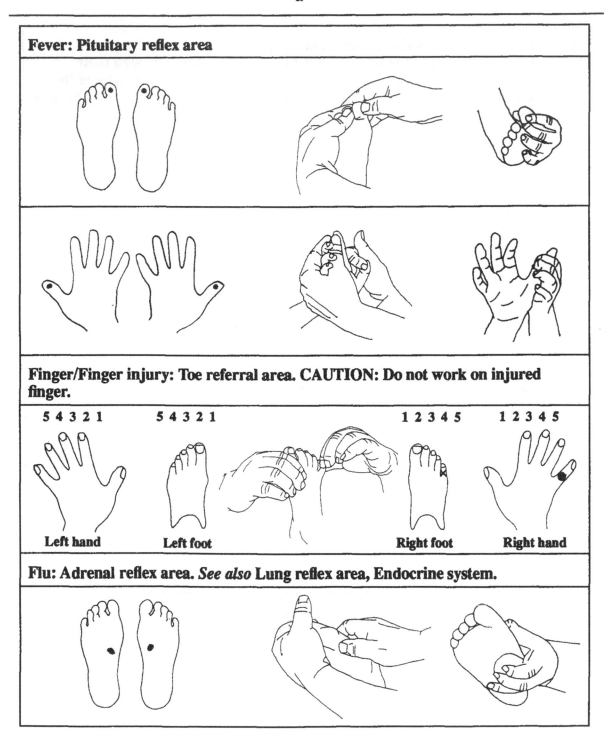

Finger/Finger injury: Toe referral area. CAUTION: Do not work on injured finger.

5 4 3 2 1   5 4 3 2 1   1 2 3 4 5   1 2 3 4 5

Left hand   Left foot   Right foot   Right hand

Flu: Adrenal reflex area. *See also* **Lung reflex area, Endocrine system.**

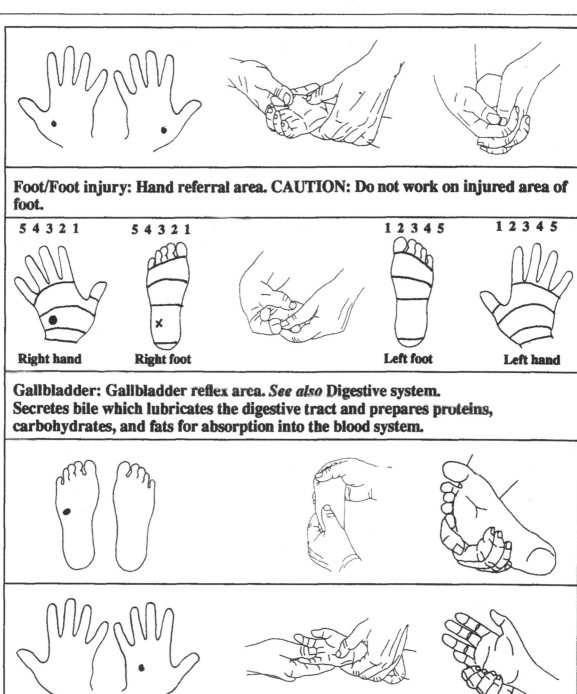

Foot/Foot injury: Hand referral area. CAUTION: Do not work on injured area of foot.

5 4 3 2 1   5 4 3 2 1   1 2 3 4 5   1 2 3 4 5

Right hand   Right foot   Left foot   Left hand

Gallbladder: Gallbladder reflex area. *See also* Digestive system.
Secretes bile which lubricates the digestive tract and prepares proteins, carbohydrates, and fats for absorption into the blood system.

Hand/Hand injury: Foot referral area. CAUTION: Do not work on injured area.

5 4 3 2 1   5 4 3 2 1   1 2 3 4 5   1 2 3 4 5

Right hand   **Right foot**   **Left foot**   **Left hand**

Hay fever: Adrenal gland reflex area. *See also* **Endocrine system.**

Head/Head injury: Head reflex area
Accommodates the brain, several sensory organs, sinus cavities, and inlets for food and air.

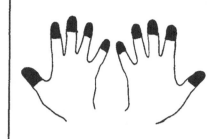 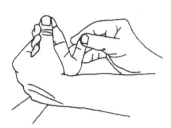 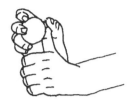

Headache: Solar plexus reflex area

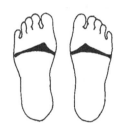 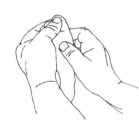 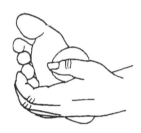

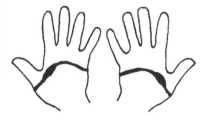 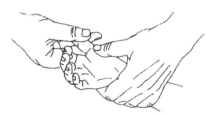 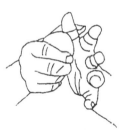

Heart: Heart reflex area. *See also* Circulatory system.
The heart is a pump whose action keeps the blood circulating, carrying nutrients, hormones, vitamins, antibodies, heat, and oxygen to the tissues, and taking waste materials away.

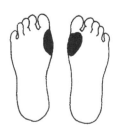 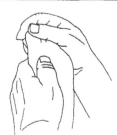 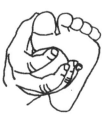

(continued on next page)

(Heart, continued)

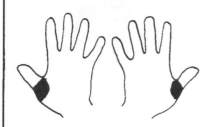 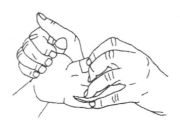 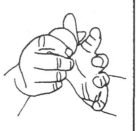

Hip/Sciatica: Hip/Sciatic reflex area

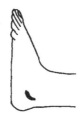 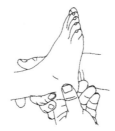 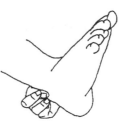

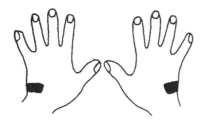 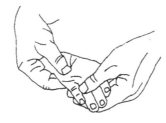 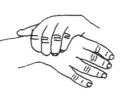

Hyperactivity: Adrenal gland reflex area. *See also* Endocrine system.

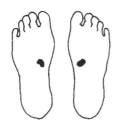 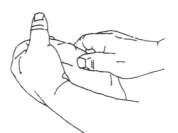 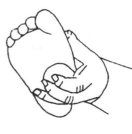

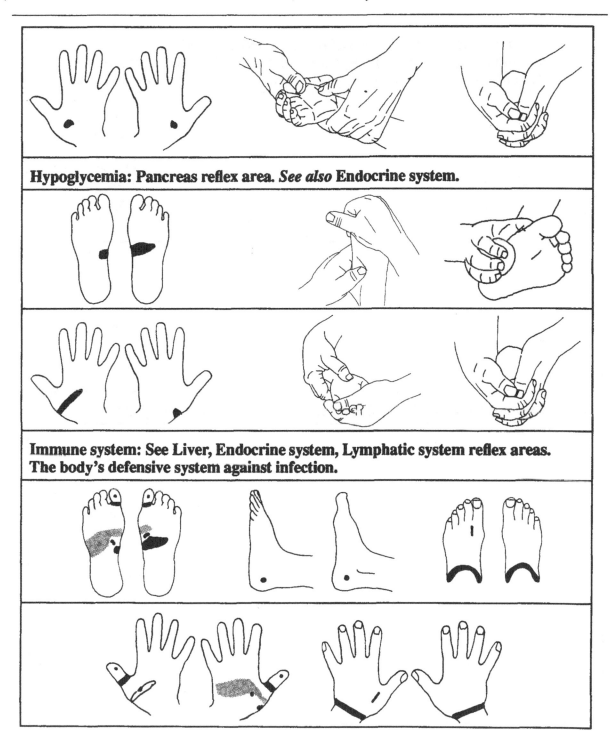

Hypoglycemia: Pancreas reflex area. *See also* Endocrine system.

Immune system: See Liver, Endocrine system, Lymphatic system reflex areas. The body's defensive system against infection.

Kidneys/Kidney infection: Kidney reflex area/Adrenal gland reflex area
Regulate fluid and purify blood: regulate acid/alkaline balance, stimulate
production of red blood cells, and regulate salt and other substances in the blood.

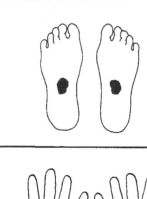 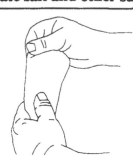 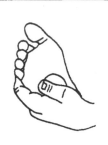

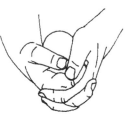

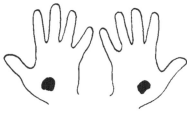 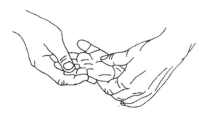 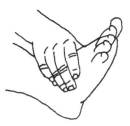

Knee/Knee injury: Knee/Leg reflex area. *See also* **Referral areas, p. 91.**

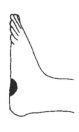 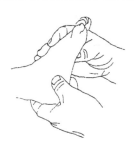 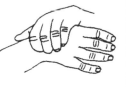

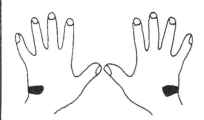 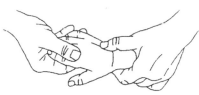

Leg/Leg injury: Knee/Leg reflex area. *See also* **Referral areas, p. 91.**

Liver: Liver reflex area. *See also* Digestive system.
Detoxifies consumed food and fluids. Stores glycogen to supply a steady concentration of fuel.

Lungs/Chest/Breast: Lung/Chest/Breast reflex area.
Regulate intake of oxygen into the blood system.

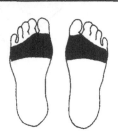 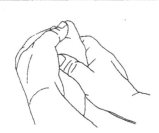 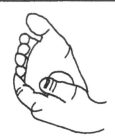

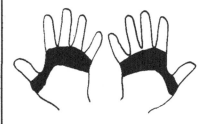 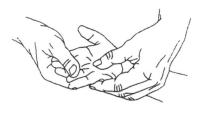 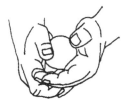

Lymphatic system: Lymphatic system reflex areas
Overall body network that filters body fluids, fights infection, and removes waste.

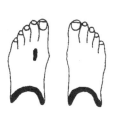 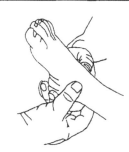 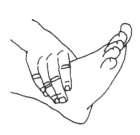

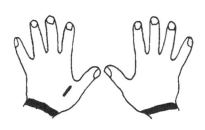 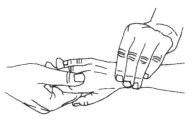 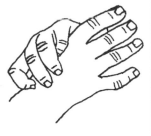

Menstruation: Uterus reflex area

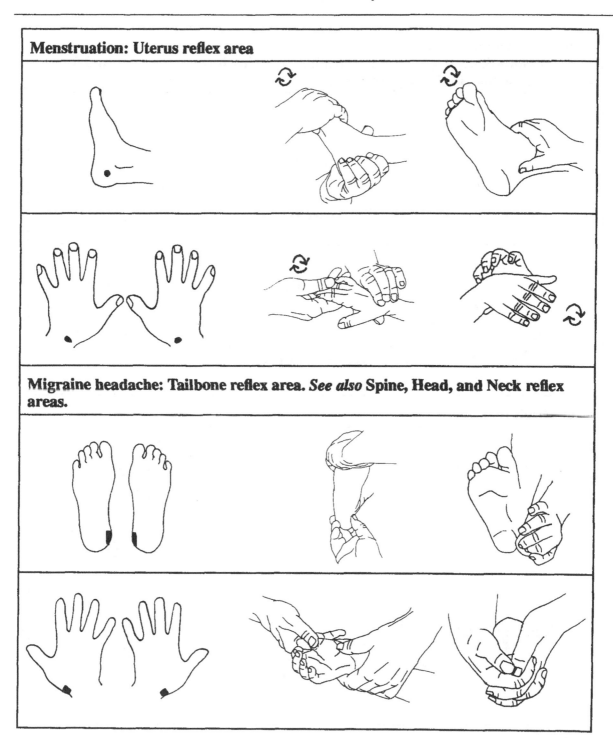

Migraine headache: Tailbone reflex area. *See also* **Spine, Head, and Neck reflex areas.**

Musculo–skeletal system
The musculo–skeletal system is responsible for giving form to the body and for providing movement. It keeps us upright.

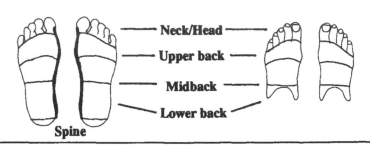

Neck/Head — Upper back — Midback — Lower back
Spine

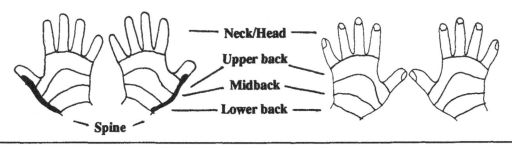

Neck/Head — Upper back — Midback — Lower back
Spine

Neck: Neck reflex area

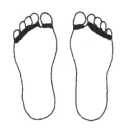
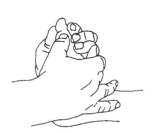
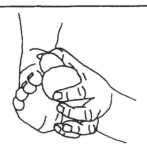

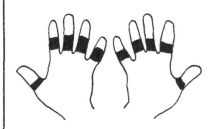
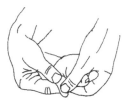
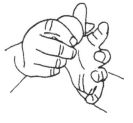

Nervous system

Regulates muscular and secretory activities of the body. Functions include the gathering of information and the response to it as well as adjustments within the internal environment. The central nervous system consists of the brain and spinal cord and the nerves emanating from them.

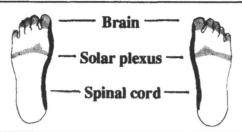

Brain —
— Solar plexus —
— Spinal cord —

Brain —
Solar plexus —
Spinal cord —
— Brain
— Solar plexus
Spinal cord

Ovary/Testicle: Ovary/Testicle reflex area. *See also* **Reproductive system. Produce hormones that influence mental vigor, physical development, and reproductive capacities. Maintain sexual urges.**

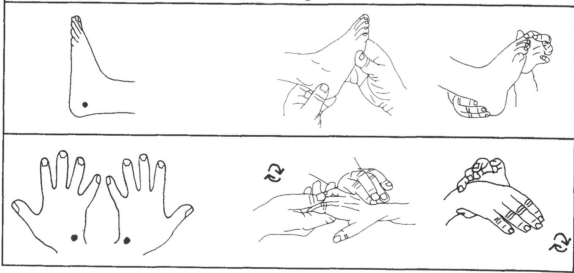

Pancreas: Pancreas reflex area. *See also* Endocrine system.
Produces a hormone that regulates blood sugar level. Produces digestive juices.

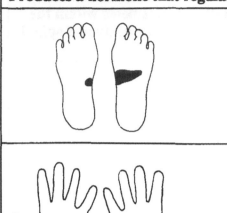 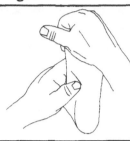 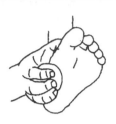

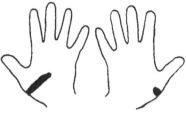 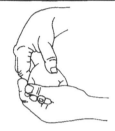 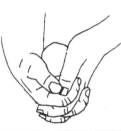

Pituitary: Pituitary reflex area. *See also* Endocrine system.
Regulates the other endocrine glands, the arteries of the heart and body, water balance, blood pressure, sexual maturation, reproduction, growth, and metabolism.

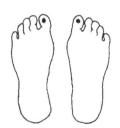 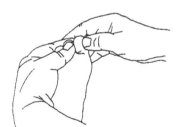 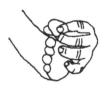

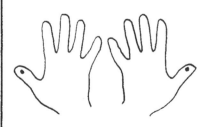 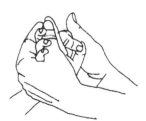 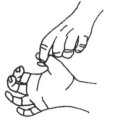

Reproductive system: Reproductive system reflex areas
Produces hormones that influence mental vigor, physical development, and reproductive capacities. Maintains sexual urge.

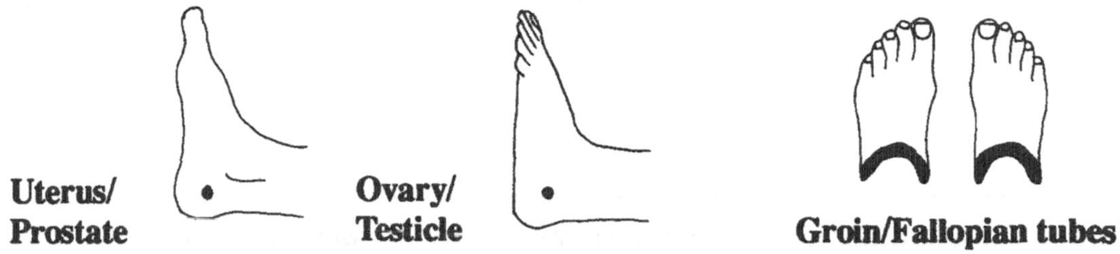

Uterus/
Prostate   Ovary/
                            Testicle   Groin/Fallopian tubes

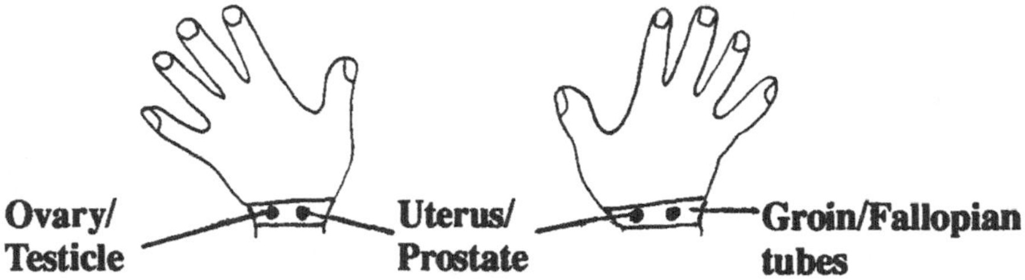

Ovary/   Uterus/   Groin/Fallopian
Testicle   Prostate   tubes

Respiratory system: Respiratory system reflex areas
Regulates intake of oxygen into the bloodstream.

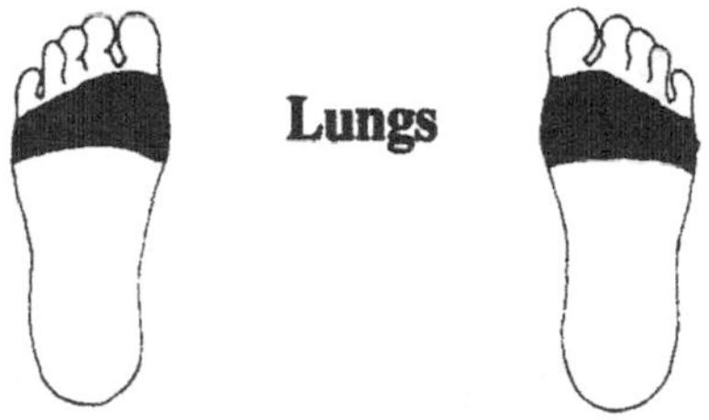

Lungs

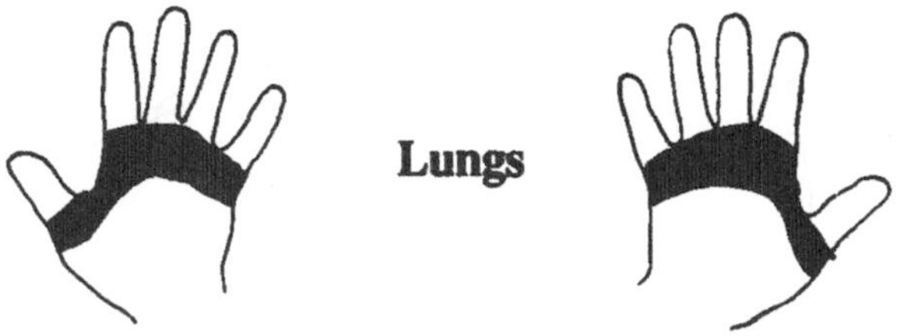

Lungs

Revival: Pituitary reflex area

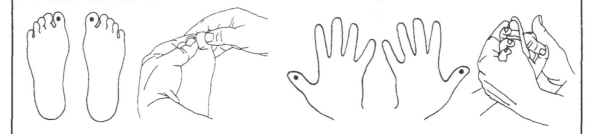

Shoulder/Shoulder injury: Shoulder reflex area. *See also* **Referral areas, p. 91.**

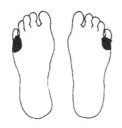 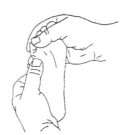 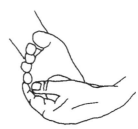

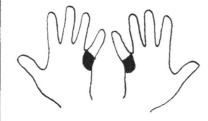 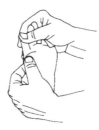 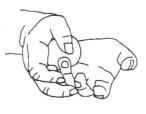

Sinus headache/infection: Adrenal gland reflex area. *See also* **Head reflex area.**

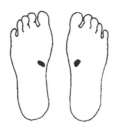 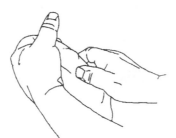 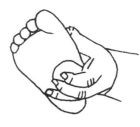

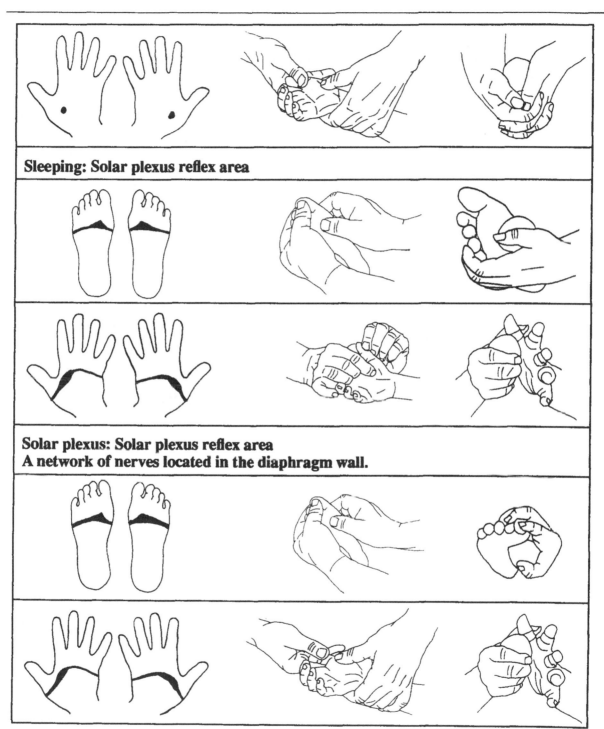

Sleeping: Solar plexus reflex area

Solar plexus: Solar plexus reflex area
A network of nerves located in the diaphragm wall.

Spleen: Spleen reflex area
Produces antibodies and filters lymph fluids. Removes and destroys faulty red blood cells and recycles iron for haemoglobin production.

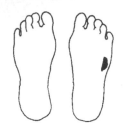 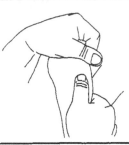 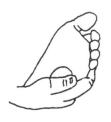

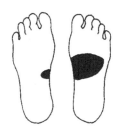 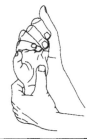 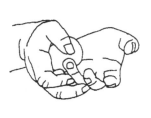

Stomach/Stomach ache: Stomach reflex area. *See also* Digestive system.
Digestion of food.

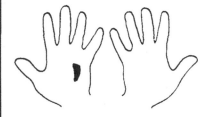 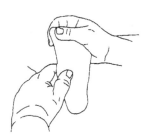 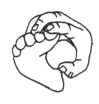

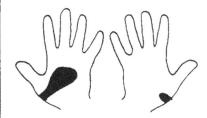 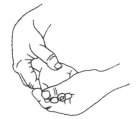 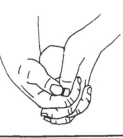

Stress: Solar plexus reflex area

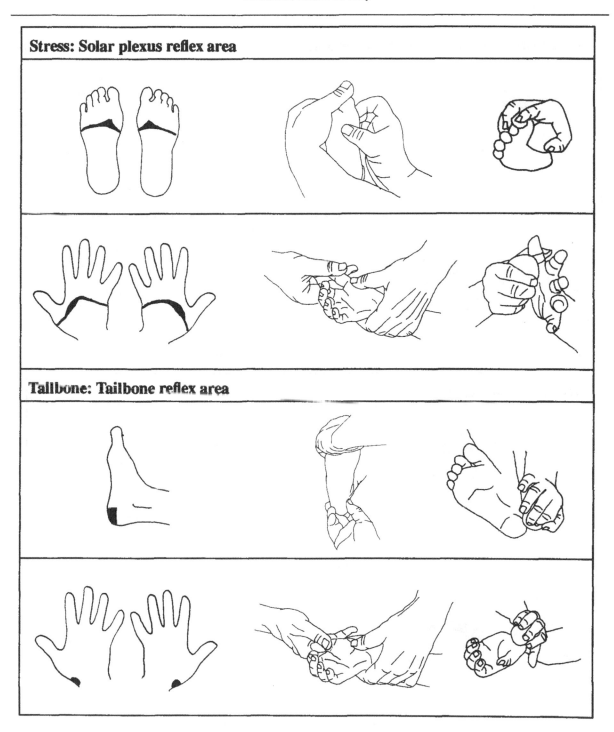

Tailbone: Tailbone reflex area

Teeth/Jaw/Teething: Teeth/jaw reflex area

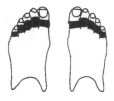
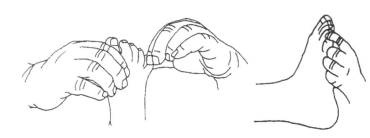

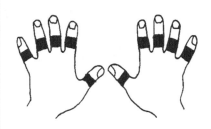
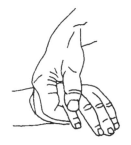
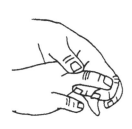

Throat: Throat reflex area

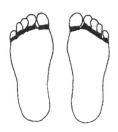
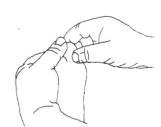
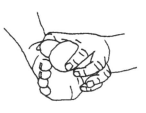

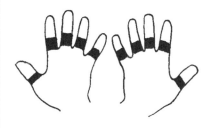
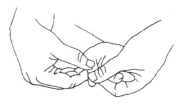
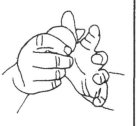

144

Thyroid/Parathyroid: Thyroid reflex area. *See also* **Endocrine system. Regulates metabolism, growth, and development. Controls calcium levels. Parathyroid glands control levels of calcium and phosphorus.**

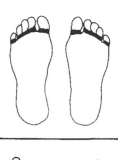 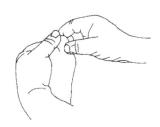 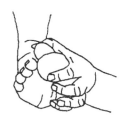

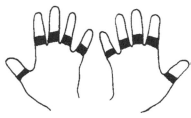 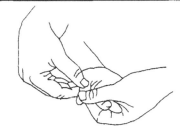 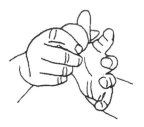

Toe/Toe injury: Finger referral area. CAUTION: Do not work on injured toe.

5 4 3 2 1   5 4 3 2 1   1 2 3 4 5   1 2 3 4 5

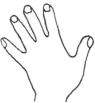 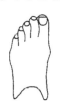 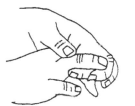 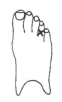 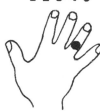

Left hand   Left foot   Right foot   Right hand

Tonsillitis: Throat reflex area. *See also* **Adrenal gland reflex area.**

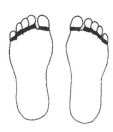 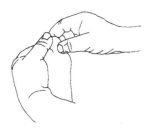 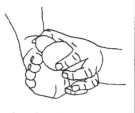

(continued on next page)

(Tonsillitis, continued)

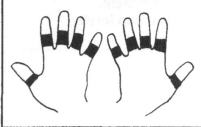 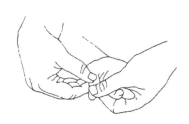 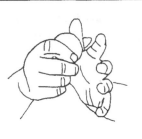

Uterus/Prostate: Uterus/Prostate reflex area. *See also* **Reproductive system. Produces hormones that influence mental vigor, physical development, and reproductive capacities. Maintain sexual urge.**

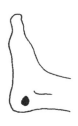 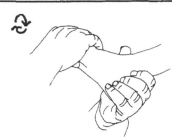 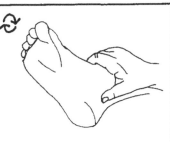

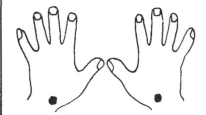 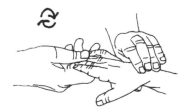 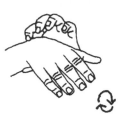

Wrist/Wrist injury: Ankle referral area. CAUTION: Do not work on injured wrist.

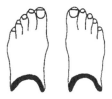 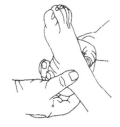 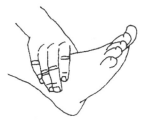

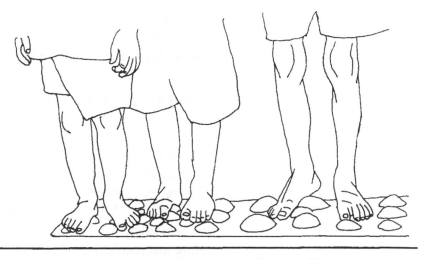

Chapter 7   Special Uses of Reflexology

Children's lives include special challenges. Reflexology provides the parent with the opportunity to take positive action to promote the child's well-being and to cope with situations that commonly arise.

The feet and hands are sensory organs — exposing them to as much variety as possible makes them a contributor to healthful development and living. Think about what the child's foot or hand goes through in a day. The challenge of learning to walk, to write, to wear shoes on hard surfaces, overuse the video game, playing sports and much more are all a part of the stress of a day which can be made easier with reflexology.

Growing Up with Reflexology

Reflexology can be used as a tool for parents or the child's significant adults to use to handle and dissipate the stresses of everyday life in a healthy way. Reflexology provides a tool chest of techniques to apply in stress-proofing the child and an opportunity to add a nutrient in helping the child to grow.

Development of a stress cue system

Some children are born with stress cues evident in their feet and hands. Others seemingly have none. For all, however, the exploration of his or her universe soon begins for the child. A full range of experiences ensues — many happy ones and a few bumps and bruises — twisting an ankle at gymnastics lessons, that allergy problem that runs in the family, the fall while skating that resulted in possibly injuring the tailbone. The application of reflexology's techniques interrupts the stress of the event. It also allows the body to make the best possible adaptation to the stress.

Reflexology can become a part of the nurturing experience. Reflexive responses—such as locomotion, alertness, and body awareness—can be influenced through reflexology techniques.

Observation of the foot

As noted previously, you will develop the skill to assess what you feel under your thumb or finger as pressure is applied to the foot or hand. By observing what you feel in the child's foot or hand, you can compare and contrast this to what you feel in other feet or hands. And you can note the changes that take place.

Health history

Another advantage to growing up with reflexology is the opportunity it provides to stay in touch with a child's health history as it unfolds. Nobody follows a child's health like a parent. I asked a twelve-year-old boy if his stomach ever bothered him. He said no. His mother then reminded him that he was always complaining about his stomach.

Reflexology is a tool to track and respond to the demands of growing up. By noting stressors and stress patterns, and writing them down, you can more effectively chart your child's physical progression. Children can be trained as well to note their bumps and bangs. How frequently does Johnny or Susie get sick? Is it every winter? Is it always lung oriented? Does the spring allergy season seem bothersome?

The family tree

"(He or she) has her daddy's (mommy's) feet." As a reflexologist, this is a phrase I hear frequently when talking about children. We all generally accept the notion that health traits run in the family. Reflexology has been utilized to respond to concerns about hereditary problems. The great-grandmother who used reflexology with her granddaughter to avert a hereditary hearing problem is an example.

Working with Self-Help Reflexology

Just as other life skills are passed along by parents, reflexology techniques are a skill worth teaching. Our niece grew up observing reflexology's technique application. She was surprised that we were surprised by her continuing use of reflexology work. A golf ball accompanied her into the delivery room. She gave birth so quickly that the hospital staff had a hard time believing that it was her first child.

Within the reflexology model, technique application breaks the cycle of stress. Further technique application creates conditioning. The ideal is thus self-help technique application. Who better than the child can perceive his or her "owies"?

Younger children especially are great mimics. To encourage the child to use self-help techniques, use self-help techniques yourself. The five-year-old with the migraine headaches mentioned earlier picked up the golf ball by himself after seeing adults use one.

The golf ball self-help technique

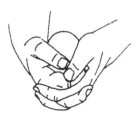

The golf ball is a simple, inexpensive self-help tool. To try using the golf ball to apply reflexology techniques, begin by holding a golf ball in your hand. Clasp your hands together, interlinking the fingers. Roll the golf ball over the palms of the hands. Press the palm of the hand below the thumb. Press the heel of the hand. Experiment also trying to achieve a result. For example, when your stomach is upset or your allergies are active, try the golf ball self-help technique. This experience will help you to provide direction to child and self-help.

If you're ever without a golf ball, a simple technique to work the hand is the single finger grip. Place your index finger tip on the palm of the hand. Exert pressure.

The natural foot

The world is not flat, but most feet wouldn't know that. Encased in shoes and walking on flat, paved surfaces, the feet do not get a chance to experience the three-dimensionality of the world.

This idea has been further explored in the Far East through the use of pathways for bare feet. The pathway underfoot consists of pebbles, embedded rocks, logs, and varied surfaces to stimulate the sole of the foot. These health pathways of Japan are designed to specifically exercise every part of the foot.

On a more practical level, simply walking on sand at the beach or a rock path provides much needed stimulation for the feet. Although commercially made products are available, common items from around the house will work as well — the handle of a broom, the rounded concrete lawn edger, rocks, wooden beads, dried peas in a box, rocks in socks, door mat, knotted jute and, dowel sticks or other cylindrical objects.

Of Special Interest

Newborns / Infants

Newborns exposed to massage will come to stick their feet and hands out to receive technique application. A child's feet grow rapidly during the first year of life. Chiropodists advise that parents take steps to help normal development. The infant should be covered loosely to enable freedom of movement or not covered at all at times to allow an opportunity to kick. In addition, lying too long, especially on the stomach, can put excessive strain on the legs and feet. Children should not be forced into shoes when starting to walk. Going barefoot or clad only in socks helps the foot to grow normally and to develop the grasping action of the toes.

Puberty

Growing pains and emotional swings are familiar to most parents of teenage children. Reflexology technique application helps to ease pain and prompts the body to undergo hormonal changes more easily. The endocrine system reflex areas are targeted for this purpose.

Sports

Mothers frequently express concern about injuries their sons experience on the playing fields. In addition to addressing concerns about injury, a recent Chinese study has demonstrated the ability of reflexology technique application to help adult athletes rebound from the fatigue of athletic competition.

Traveling with children

Challenges to parents traveling with children include boredom, stress, and physical discomfort. An arsenal of reflexology techniques can help entertain and soothe the restless child.

A reflexology workout can keep children calmer. A few presses to the solar plexus reflex area of the hand can help if there is no opportunity for a full workout.

Showing the child self-help techniques to apply can keep him or her busy. For example, does the child's back hurt from sitting in one place too long? Show him or her where to work on the hand and then create the game of seeing how long it takes to make the back pain go away.

Travel can be physically discomforting for anyone. Young children commonly experience pain in the ears during take-offs and landings while traveling by plane. When the plane took off, our niece's hands went to her infant's feet and his ear reflex area. She notes that frequently her baby is the only one on the airplane not crying during takeoff and landing.

Working with the Special Child

A special child provides unique challenges to parents. Reflexology can be utilized both formally and informally to meet these challenges.

Informally, one mother told us that she used reflexology to address the side issues associated with her son's Downs syndrome. Another mother sought to improve her son's ability to walk, which was slightly impaired by cerebral palsy.

Formally, centers in Scotland and the United States utilize reflexology as a part of programs for brain injured children. It is used as a form of sensory-motor exercise to help rebuild the injured nervous system. (For information, write Society for the Advancement of Brain Injured Children, David Elder Centre, 503 Langlands Road, Govan, Glasgow, Scotland G51 4JY.)

Reflex areas targeted in general with the special child include the nervous system and endocrine glands which control the activities of the body. Reflex areas include brain, spinal cord, solar plexus, eye/ear, and endocrine glands.

Pressure techniques application may provoke spasms of the legs. It may even be difficult or impossible to work with the feet because of this. Apply technique to the hand if application to the foot is difficult or impossible. Over time, spasms should diminish as a response to pressure technique application.

Condition	Technique Application
Brain injury	Apply pressure to brain (big toe) and spine reflex areas. Find areas of special emphasis in the big toe for further technique application by noting what you feel under your thumb. NOTE: Application of pressure to the feet may prompt a response of spasming into a rigid position. If the spasm makes works impossible, try working with the hand.
Cerebral palsy	Apply pressure to the solar plexus, brain, and spine reflex areas.
Downs syndrome	Apply pressure techniques to the brain and spine reflex areas.
Hyperactivity	Apply pressure techniques to the pancreas, adrenal gland, and brain reflex areas.
Learning difficulties	Apply pressure techniques to the brain and spine reflex areas.
Multiple sclerosis	Apply pressure techniques to the brain and spine reflex areas. Find areas of special emphasis in the spinal reflex area for further technique application by noting what you feel under your thumb.
Paralysis	Apply pressure to the spine, eye/ear, kidney, and bladder reflex areas. Find areas of special emphasis in the spine reflex area for further technique application by noting what you feel under your thumb. Try to find the mirror image area of the spinal injury if paralysis is due to a spinal cord injury. NOTE: Spasms with movement is a common response to the application of pressure. Note the part of the foot that triggers the response. It is an area for special emphasis. Apply technique lightly, increasing pressure over time.

Resources

Finding a reflexologist

Call the reflexologist and interview him or her. Ask questions about education, credentials, years of experience, and experience working with children. Next try a sample session yourself or for the child.

Consider your goal in seeking the services of a reflexologist. Are you interested in having a specialist apply a completed session of reflexology techniques? Are you seeking to use the practitioner's services as an adjunct to your own reflexology work with your child? A reflexologist is a specialist who knows how deeply, where, and in what pattern to apply technique. His or her work can provide a brief education for you about your work with your child.

The Association of Reflexologists, 27 Old Gloucester Street, London WC1 3XX maintains a directory of practitioners.

Taking classes

The Association of Reflexologists, 27 Old Gloucester Street, London WC1 3XX maintains a list of accredited schools.

Reference books

Kunz, Kevin and Barbara Kunz, *The Complete Guide to Foot Reflexology*, London, Thorsons, 1984.

Kunz, Kevin and Barbara Kunz, *Hand and Foot Reflexology, A Self-Help Guide*, London, Thorsons, 1984.

Index

Hand Reflexology Chart

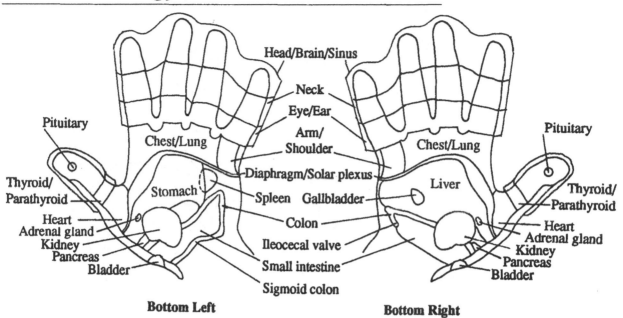

Bottom Left

Bottom Right

Head/Brain/Sinus
Neck
Eye/Ear
Arm/Shoulder
Diaphragm/Solar plexus
Spleen   Gallbladder
Colon
Ileocecal valve
Small intestine
Sigmoid colon

Pituitary
Chest/Lung
Stomach

Thyroid/Parathyroid
Heart
Adrenal gland
Kidney
Pancreas
Bladder

Liver
Chest/Lung
Pituitary
Thyroid/Parathyroid
Heart
Adrenal gland
Kidney
Pancreas
Bladder

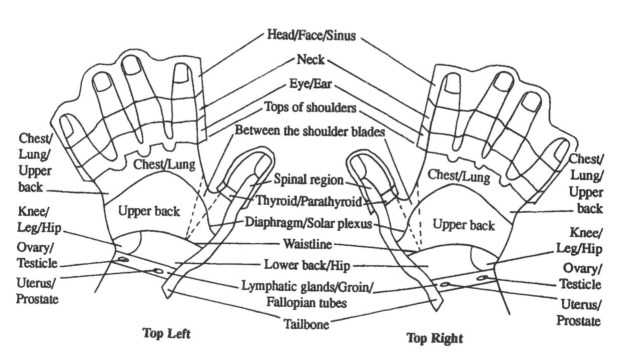

Top Left

Top Right

Head/Face/Sinus
Neck
Eye/Ear
Tops of shoulders
Between the shoulder blades
Spinal region
Thyroid/Parathyroid
Diaphragm/Solar plexus
Waistline
Lower back/Hip
Lymphatic glands/Groin/Fallopian tubes
Tailbone

Chest/Lung/Upper back
Chest/Lung
Upper back
Knee/Leg/Hip
Ovary/Testicle
Uterus/Prostate

Chest/Lung
Upper back
Chest/Lung/Upper back
Knee/Leg/Hip
Ovary/Testicle
Uterus/Prostate

157

Foot Reflexology Chart

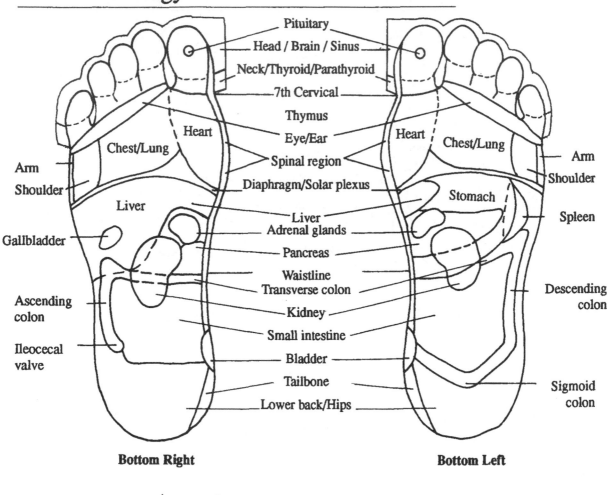

Bottom Right

Bottom Left

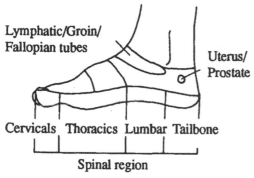

Inside Right

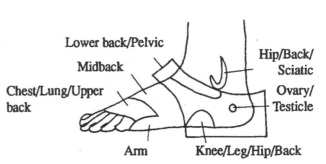

Outside Left

158

CPSIA information can be obtained at www.ICGtesting.com
Printed in the USA
LVOW021642140413

329061LV00005B/248/P